Emergency Care and First Aid for Nurses

For Elsevier:

Commissioning Editor: **Steven Black**
Development Editor: **Catherine Jackson**
Project Manager: **Gail Wright**
Designer: **Stewart Larking**
Illustration Buyer: **Gillian Murray**
Illustrator: **Cactus & Chartwell**

Emergency Care
and First Aid for Nurses

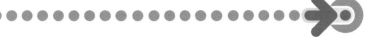

A PRACTICAL GUIDE

Philip Jevon RN BSc(Hons) PGCE
Resuscitation Council (UK) ALS EPLS NLS Instructor
Resuscitation Officer/Clinical Skills Lead, Manor Hospital,
Walsall, UK

Consultant Editors

David F. Bowden FRCS FFAEM
Consultant in Emergency Medicine, Accident and Emergency
Department, Good Hope Hospital, Sutton Coldfield, UK

David Halliwell MSc State Registered Paramedic
Resuscitation Council Instructor; Head of Education and
Professional Development, Dorset Ambulance NHS Trust,
Bournemouth, UK

Robin M. McMahon SBStJ BSc RGN RSCN FAETC
Advanced Neonatal Nurse Practitioner, Neonatal Intensive Care
Unit, New Cross Hospital, Wolverhampton, UK

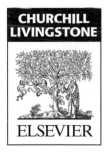

CHURCHILL
LIVINGSTONE

ELSEVIER

EDINBURGH LONDON NEW YORK OXFORD PHILADELPHIA ST LOUIS SYDNEY TORONTO 2007

CHURCHILL
LIVINGSTONE
ELSEVIER

© 2007, Elsevier Limited. All rights reserved.

First published 2007

ISBN-13: 978-0-443-10208-0
ISBN-10: 0 443 10208 2

British Library Cataloguing in Publication Data
A catalogue record for this book is available from the British Library.

Library of Congress Cataloging in Publication Data
A catalog record for this book is available from the Library of Congress.

Note
Knowledge and best practice in this field are constantly changing. As new research and experience broaden our knowledge, changes in practice, treatment and drug therapy may become necessary or appropriate. Readers are advised to check the most current information provided (i) on procedures featured or (ii) by the manufacturer of each product to be administered, to verify the recommended dose or formula, the method and duration of administration, and contraindications. It is the responsibility of the practitioner, relying on their own experience and knowledge of the patient, to make diagnoses, to determine dosages and the best treatment for each individual patient, and to take all appropriate safety precautions. To the fullest extent of the law, neither the Publisher nor the Authors assume any liability for any injury and/or damage to persons or property arising out of, or related to, any use of the material contained in this book.

The Publisher

ELSEVIER your source for books,
journals and multimedia
in the health sciences
www.elsevierhealth.com

Working together to grow
libraries in developing countries
www.elsevier.com | www.bookaid.org | www.sabre.org

ELSEVIER   BOOK AID   Sabre Foundation
            International

Printed in China

Contents

Contributors

Bridgit Dimond MA LLB DSA AHSM Barrister-at-Law
Emeritus Professor, University of Glamorgan, UK
Chapter 21 – Legal aspects of first aid

Mark Gillett BSc(Hons) MBBS FRCS(A&E) FFAEM FFSEM
MSc DipIMCRCSEd
Consultant and Clinical Director, Emergency Medicine, Good
Hope NHS Trust, Good Hope Hospital, Sutton Coldfield, UK
Chapter 15 – Musculoskeletal injuries

Acknowledgements

I am grateful to Avril Morgan, Epilepsy Nurse Specialist, Manor Hospital Walsall, for her advice on the first aid treatment during a seizure; to Dr Kathleen Berry, Consultant Paediatrician, A & E, Birmingham Children's Hospital, for her help with the paediatric content of the book; to Denise Fraser, Matron A & E, Manor Hospital Walsall, for her help and advice with some of the images; and to John Hamilton, Medical Photography, Manor Hospital Walsall, for his help with some of the images.

First aid:
an overview

First aid: an overview

Introduction

First aid can be defined as 'the initial assistance or treatment given to someone who is injured or suddenly taken ill' (St John Ambulance, 2002). It can cover a wide range of scenarios ranging from simple reassurance following a minor mishap to dealing with a life-threatening emergency.

Providing first aid can be very stressful; the stress of working in unfamiliar circumstances, sometimes with inquisitive and intrusive onlookers, should not be underestimated. It is important to remain calm and focused on the priorities.

The aim of this chapter is to provide an overview to first aid.

Chapter objectives
At the end of the chapter the reader will be able to:

- List the priorities of first aid

- Discuss the responsibilities when providing first aid

- Outline the assessment of the casualty

- State the procedure for alerting the emergency services

- Discuss the methods to reduce the risk of cross-infection

- Describe the environmental hazards that may be encountered

- Discuss the provision of first aid at road traffic accidents

- Outline the principles of first aid at road traffic accidents

- Discuss the NMC's guidelines on nurses providing first aid

Priorities of first aid

The priorities of first aid are to:

- ensure the appropriate emergency services are alerted
- ensure both the rescuer and casualty's safety
- keep the casualty alive: attention to airway, breathing and circulation is paramount
- prevent the casualty from deteriorating
- promote the recovery of the casualty
- provide reassurance and comfort to the casualty.

Responsibilities when providing first aid

Although the provision of first aid is not an exact science, it is important to remember the golden rule: 'first do no harm', while applying the term 'calculated risk' (St John Ambulance, 2002). When providing first aid, nurses have a number of responsibilities including:

- assessing the situation quickly and safely
- ensuring appropriate help is summoned
- protecting the casualty and others at the scene from possible harm
- identifying as far as possible the cause of the illness or the nature of the injury
- providing first aid within their own sphere of expertise and competence
- ensuring that any first aid provided follows current and up-to-date guidelines where appropriate
- minimising the risk of cross-infection
- reporting observations/findings to those taking over the care of the casualty
- adhering to the NMC's Code of Professional Conduct (2003)
- maintaining the casualty's confidentiality following NMC's guidelines
- obtaining the casualty's consent (if possible) prior to administering first aid.

Assessment of the casualty

Safe approach

The initial priority is always to check for any dangers. Approach the casualty carefully, ensuring there is no danger, either to the rescuer or the casualty: look out for hazards, e.g. electricity, fire and traffic. Measures to minimise the risk of cross-infection should be considered (see below).

Primary survey

The priority is then to assess the casualty for life-threatening conditions and provide life-saving treatment as required. This phase, often referred to as the primary survey, involves assessing:
- Airway
- Breathing
- Circulation
- Disability
- Exposure.

Secondary survey

Once it is established that the casualty is out of immediate danger, perform a secondary survey. Depending on the situation, this could involve:
- taking a history
- looking for external clues
- ascertaining the mechanics of injury
- assessing signs and symptoms
- head to toe survey (St John Ambulance, 2002).

Definitive care

Depending on the scenario, definitive care could involve:
- providing advice only
- advising the casualty to visit a GP
- arranging transport to take the casualty to hospital
- alerting the emergency services.

Procedure for alerting the emergency services

Dial 999 (or 112) to alert the emergency services and request the service required (usually ambulance). The following information is essential:
- name of person making telephone call
- telephone number of phone from which call is being made
- exact location of the incident or problem; road name or number and if possible include any specific landmark or junction nearby
- time of the incident
- exact details of the incident; if it is relevant the number of casualties, their age and sex and any information known about their condition
- details of any casualties trapped
- details of any hazards, e.g. gas, toxic substances, damage to power-lines.

Measures to minimise the risk of cross-infection

Measures to minimise the risk of cross-infection should be taken. Simple measures, such as hand-washing and the wearing of disposable gloves, can be very effective at preventing cross-infection.

Blood is the single most important source of the transmission of HIV and hepatitis B virus. Universal precautions should apply to blood, semen, vaginal secretions and cerebrospinal, synovial, pleural, peritoneal, pericardial and amniotic fluids and any body fluid containing visible blood. Care with sharps is paramount as both HIV and the hepatitis B virus have been contracted by healthcare workers following needle-stick injuries (Marcus, 1988).

Cross-infection during mouth-to-mouth ventilation is a particular concern. Both healthcare workers and laypersons are often reluctant to perform mouth-to-mouth ventilation, most commonly due to a fear of contracting HIV. However, there have only been 15 documented cases of the transmission of infection through mouth-to-mouth ventilation, none of which involved HIV or hepatitis B virus (Mejicano & Maki, 1998). However, the re-emergence of tuberculosis is a cause for concern, particularly as it can be transmitted through mouth-to-mouth ventilation.

There is a theoretical risk of the transmission of HIV and hepatitis B during mouth-to-mouth ventilation in cases of facial trauma, or if there are breaks in the skin around the lips or soft tissues of the oral cavity mucosa (Piazza et al, 1989). Caution is particularly warranted in these situations. In a cardiac arrest, if it is impossible or ill-advised to provide mouth-to-mouth ventilation, give chest compressions only at a rate of 100/min (Resuscitation Council UK, 2005).

There is a variety of barrier devices available; facemasks with one-way valves prevent the transmission of bacteria, while face shields are less effective (Centers for Disease Control, 1991).

Environmental hazards that may be encountered

There are a number of environmental hazards that may be encountered when providing first aid, including hazardous substances, gas, electricity, fire and poisoning.

Hazardous substances

At the scene of a road traffic accident, look out for any Hazchem placards on vehicles (Fig. 1.1). Particular care should be taken if

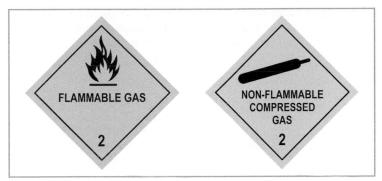

Figure 1.1 Hazchem placards

there is a letter 'E' in the top left panel of the placard, as it signifies a public safety hazard. Exposure to spillages of hazardous substances or the escaping toxic gases could pose a significant risk to the rescuer and bystanders; inform the emergency services, remain away from the scene and remain up-wind of the hazard.

Gas

If there is a smell of gas or a gas leak is detected, if it is safe to do so switch off the gas supply at the control valve, which is usually located next to the gas meter. Then:

- open doors and windows to disperse the gas
- check to see if the gas supply to an appliance has been left on, unlit or if the pilot light has gone out
- do not smoke, use matches or naked flames
- do not turn electrical switches on or off – this includes the door bell
- ensure Transco are informed of the gas leak – 0800 111 999 (London Energy, 2004).

Low voltage electricity

Injuries caused by electricity often occur in the home environment as a result of contact with a low-voltage domestic current, usually due to a faulty switch or appliance. The presence of water introduces additional risks. The electrical contact needs to be broken (British Red Cross, 2003).

Do not touch the casualty if still in contact with the electrical current. Switch off the current at the mains or meter point if it can be easily reached; otherwise remove the plug or wrench the cable free. If unable to reach the plug, cable or mains:

- stand on some dry insulating material, e.g. telephone directory, wooden box
- using a wooden object, e.g. broom, push the casualty's limbs away from the electrical source or push the latter away from the casualty (Fig. 1.2). Do not use anything metallic
- if the casualty still remains attached to the electrical current, carefully loop some rope around his ankles and pull him away from the source (British Red Cross, 2003).

Whatever is used to disconnect the casualty from the electrical source, it should be dry and non-conducting (Scottish & Southern Energy, 2001).

High voltage electricity

The Electricity Association (2004) has issued basic guidance when attempting to rescue a casualty in the vicinity of high voltage electricity. Some key points to note:

- electrical equipment can carry power ranging from 230V to 40 000V – even 230V can be fatal
- touching electrical conductors or objects/persons in contact with electrical conductors can be fatal

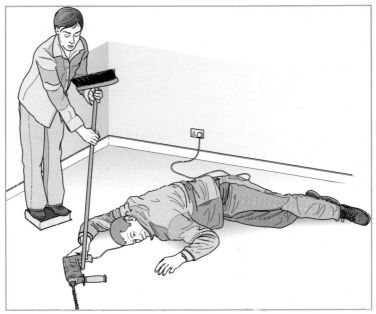

Figure 1.2 Disconnecting a casualty in contact with low voltage electrical current: use a wooden object

- trees, rope, string, fences, water and road crash barriers can conduct electricity
- electricity can jump gaps – arcing up to 5 metres
- rubber shoes will not protect the rescuer
- emergency contact telephone number for the Electrical Company is clearly displayed on notices at substation gates and most towers
- an electrical circuit may automatically be switched back on at any time (Electricity Association, 2004).

If in doubt keep at least 5 metres away and await advice from the electrical company (Electricity Association, 2004).

Treatment

- Alert the emergency services
- Contact the electrical company regarding shutting off the power
- Do not approach the casualty or allow anyone else to do so until the electrical company has confirmed it is safe to do so – high voltage electricity can arc up to 5 metres
- Once it is safe to do so, assess the casualty and start CPR if required. Contact with high voltage electricity is usually fatal (British Red Cross, 2003)

Fire

The British Red Cross (2003) recommends the following:
- raise the alarm: activate the nearest fire alarm and warn people who are at risk; call the fire and rescue services
- assess for danger: if the fire is small, is discovered early and a fire blanket or appropriate fire extinguisher is available, try to smother the flames; if unable to extinguish the flames within 30 seconds leave the building
- get to safety: leave the building and close doors behind you; do not enter a smoke-filled room; follow fire escape route if appropriate.

Some basic principles:
- don't use an elevator – if the electricity fails the elevator may abruptly stop working; also the elevator shaft can act like a chimney, sucking up flames and fumes
- if in a room full of smoke, remain close to the floor and if possible cover the nose and mouth with a damp cloth or towel
- close doors on a fire
- never open a door that is hot or has hot handles – suggests that a fire is raging behind it
- if unable to find an escape route, locate a fire-free room that has a window; shut the door, open the window and call out for help, and remain close to the floor; if possible block any gaps under the door
- even if it is dark, don't turn on the light as this may cause an explosion

- children may hide away in cupboards and wardrobes
- if clothing is on fire: stop, drop and roll:
    - Stop the casualty from running around as this can fan the flames
    - Drop him to the floor and if possible quickly wrap in a heavy fabric, e.g. woollen blanket (do not use anything synthetic)
    - Roll the casualty gently along the floor until the flames are extinguished
    (St John Ambulance, 2002; British Red Cross, 2003; Keech, 2004).

Poisoning

The casualty's exhaled air should be avoided in hydrogen cyanide or hydrogen sulphide gas poisoning. Ventilation should be undertaken using a non-return valve system. Corrosive chemicals, e.g. strong acids, alkalis or paraquat, can easily be absorbed through the skin and respiratory tract; care should be taken when handling the patient's clothes and bodily fluids, particularly vomit. Ideally, protective clothing and gloves should be worn.

Rescue from water

The majority of drowning accidents involve people who either have been swimming in strong currents or very cold water or have been swimming or boating while under the influence of alcohol (St John Ambulance, 2002). Cold water is particularly dangerous and can cause:

- uncontrollable gasping which can result in water inhalation
- a sudden rise in blood pressure which could precipitate a cardiac arrest
- a sudden inability to swim
- severe hypothermia following prolonged exposure
  (St John Ambulance, 2002).

The Royal Life Saving Society (RLSS) and the Royal Society for the Prevention of Accidents (ROSPA) (2005) have published guidelines on providing assistance to a casualty who is drowning:

- shout clear instructions to guide the casualty to safety
- direct the casualty to safety with hand signals
- reach out to the casualty with a stick, scarf, etc; to minimise the risk of being pulled into the water by the casualty, crouch or lie down (Fig. 1.3)
- throw a rope or something that will float, e.g. a ball, plastic bottle or lifebuoy, to the casualty
- if there is a boat nearby and it can be safely used, row out to the casualty.

The underlying principles are to ensure help is on the way, to assist the casualty without getting into the water and to avoid placing yourself at risk. However, it may be necessary (as long as it is safe to do so) to wade into the water, e.g. if the casualty is unconscious,

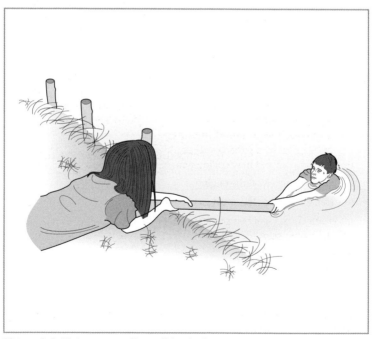

Figure 1.3 Water rescue: if possible, don't enter the water; instead reach out to the casualty with an object, e.g. a stick

or even swim out to the casualty and tow him in – **ideally, this should be undertaken by someone trained in water rescue**. If wading in, test the depth of the water using a stick or similar, carefully wade into the water and then reach out to the casualty using a stick (RLSS & ROSPA, 2005).

First aid at road traffic accidents

In the UK, road traffic accidents cause 320 000 injuries, 40 000 serious and 3400 deaths each year (World Health Organization, 2002). As road traffic accidents are very common, it is highly probable that nurses will at some time in their career encounter one. However, for those not familiar and trained to work in the pre-hospital environment, the experience can be very distressing and daunting (Coats & Davies, 2002). However, some basic principles can be helpful.

If stopping at a crash scene to offer assistance, ensure your car is parked in a safe place, ideally off the road and well clear of the incident site. It may be helpful to leave the car's hazard warning lights on. Approach with extreme care and stop and look for hazards. It is essential to ensure that it is safe to approach. Many hazards may be encountered including:

- risk of being hit by a passing vehicle; drivers of passing vehicles will be easily distracted and may collide with rescue workers or wreckage
- risk of fire – switch off the engine
- vehicles involved in the crash may be unstable
- if the vehicle has seat belt pre-tensioners and airbags (contain explosives) which haven't been activated on impact, these may be set off during extrication of the casualty
- sharp metal edges and glass
  (Coats & Davies, 2002).

The following general precautions are recommended to help make the environment safe:
- at night, wear or carry something that is bright or reflective and use a torch

- ask other bystanders to warn other drivers to slow down
- place warning triangles at least 45 metres from the incident site in each direction
- stabilise damaged vehicles; switch off the ignition and apply the handbrake; if possible disconnect the battery and also switch off the fuel supply on diesel vehicles and motorcycles if possible
- ensure nobody smokes
- look for Hazchem notices on vehicles (see Fig. 1.1); spillages of dangerous substances or the escape of toxic vapours can be particularly hazardous
- inform the emergency services if there are damaged power lines, Hazchem notices or spilt fuel.

When alerting the emergency services, the precise location of the incident is the most important information to give (by street name and intersection or junction, with the direction of travel if on a dual carriageway or motorway). If a casualty is trapped in a vehicle, it is also important to alert the fire and rescue services.

Once it is safe to approach, quickly assess all the casualties. First aid treatment should follow the familiar ABC approach, with particular attention to cervical spine immobilisation; do not move a casualty unless there is danger of further injury. Also check for casualties who may have been thrown some distance from a vehicle or may have wandered away in shock.

Conclusion

First aid can cover a wide range of scenarios ranging from simple reassurance following a minor mishap to dealing with a life-threatening emergency. Many hazards can be encountered. It is important to remain calm and focused on the priorities. An overview to the principles of providing first aid has been provided.

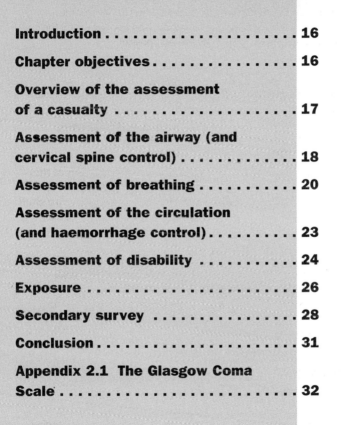

Assessment of the casualty

Introduction

Before undertaking an assessment of the casualty, the initial priority is to check for hazards (see Chapter 1). Approach the casualty carefully, ensuring there are no hazards, e.g. electricity, fire and traffic. Then assess the casualty. Initially a primary survey should be undertaken to assess for life-threatening conditions that require life-saving first aid. The comprehensiveness of the assessment required will depend on the situation. Clearly, if the casualty has collapsed and appears to be lifeless, only a simple assessment following Resuscitation Council (UK) BLS guidelines will be initially required (see Chapter 3). Once it is established that the casualty is not in immediate danger, a secondary survey should then be undertaken.

The aim of this chapter is to understand the assessment of the casualty.

Chapter objectives
At the end of the chapter the reader will be able to:

- **Detail an overview of the assessment of the casualty**

- **Describe the assessment of the airway (and cervical spine control)**

- **Describe the assessment of the breathing**

- **Describe the assessment of the circulation (and haemorrhage control)**

- **Describe the assessment of conscious level**

- **Describe procedures for removing a protective helmet**

Overview of the assessment of a casualty

When assessing the casualty, the priority is to assess the casualty for life-threatening conditions that require life-saving first aid. This phase, often referred to as the primary survey, involves assessing:

- Airway (and cervical spine control)
- Breathing
- Circulation (and haemorrhage control)
- Disability
- Exposure.

If the casualty has collapsed and appears to be lifeless, only a simple assessment, following Resuscitation Council UK guidelines (2005) is initially required. BLS can then be promptly started if required (see Chapter 3).

Once it is established that the casualty is not in immediate danger and no deficits were found duing the primary survey, a secondary survey should be performed. Depending on the situation, this could involve:

- taking a history
- looking for external clues
- ascertaining the mechanics of injury
- assessing signs and symptoms
- head to toe survey
  (St John Ambulance, 2002).

Once the casualty has been assessed, the first aid and definitive care requirements can be established. Depending on the scenario, definitive care could involve:

- providing advice only
- advising the casualty to visit a GP
- arranging transport to take the casualty to hospital
- alerting the emergency services.

Assessement of the airway (and cervical spine control)

Airway obstruction can be life-threatening. It can be partial or complete and can occur at any level of the respiratory tract from the mouth to the trachea. Causes of upper airway obstruction include:

- tongue (in a semi-conscious or unconscious casualty, the most common cause of airway obstruction is the tongue falling back and blocking the pharynx (Smith, 2003)
- vomit, blood and secretions
- foreign body
- tissue swelling (caused by allergy, trauma or infection).

Causes of lower airway obstruction include:
- laryngeal oedema (due to burns, inflammation, inflammation or allergy occurring at the level of the larynx)
- laryngeal spasm (due to foreign body, airway stimulation or secretions/blood in the airway)
- tracheobronchial obstruction (due to aspiration of gastric contents, secretions, pulmonary oedema fluid or bronchospasm) (Smith, 2003).

Assess the patency of the airway and identify the casualty's airway for signs of obstruction. Recognition of airway obstruction is based on the simple 'look, listen and feel approach'.

Look

Look for signs of airway obstruction:
- paradoxical chest and abdominal movements – see-saw respiratory pattern of the chest when there is complete airway obstruction, but the casualty is still making respiratory efforts
- use of accessory muscles of respiration (neck and abdomen) and tracheal tug

- cyanosis – central cyanosis is a late sign of airway obstruction (Smith, 2003)

Central cyanosis is a late sign of airway obstruction

Listen

Listen for signs of airway obstruction. In complete airway obstruction no breath sounds will be heard at the mouth or nose. In partial airway obstruction, although air entry is diminished, it is often noisy and certain noises help to localise the level and cause of the obstruction.

- **Inspiratory stridor**: 'croaking' sound on inspiration due to laryngeal or tracheal partial obstruction, e.g. foreign body, laryngeal oedema
- **Expiratory wheeze**: a whistling sound more pronounced on expiration; causes include asthma and chronic obstructive airways disorder
- **'Rattley' chest**: e.g. chest infection, pulmonary oedema and sputum retention
- **Gurgling**: fluid in the mouth or upper airway
- **Snoring**: caused by the tongue partially blocking the upper airway in an unconscious casualty.

Feel

Feel for signs of breathing at the mouth and nose (use face or hand).

Cervical spine control

If there is a suspicion of cervical spine injury, keep the head and neck still and in alignment (see p. 161). Causes of a cervical spine injury include head injury, road traffic accident, horse-riding accident, fall from a height, diving into shallow water and a rugby scrum accident.

If it is necessary to open the casualty's airway, lift the chin but try to avoid tilting the head.

Opening the airway is the first priority and a degree of head tilt may be unavoidable

Assessment of breathing

Recognition of respiratory distress or inadequate ventilation is based on the simple 'look, listen and feel approach' (Smith, 2003) to assess the efficacy of breathing, work of breathing and adequacy of ventilation.

Efficacy of breathing

Assess the efficacy of breathing:
- **air entry**: look, listen and feel for signs of breathing
- **chest movement**: normal chest movement should be bilateral, equal and symmetrical; unilateral chest movement suggests unilateral disease, e.g. pneumothorax and pneumonia
- **depth of breathing**: rapid shallow breathing may indicate respiratory lung disease which could lead to respiratory failure (Chestnutt & Prendergast, 2004).

Work of breathing

Assess the work of breathing. Normal breathing is quiet and accomplished with minimal effort. Signs of increased work of breathing include:
- **tachypnoea**: often the first sign of respiratory distress; normal resting respiratory rate is 12–20 per minute (bradypnoea may be an ominous sign and can be caused by drugs, e.g. opiates, fatigue, hypothermia and CNS depression)
- **accessory muscle use**: e.g. neck and abdominal muscles

- **Kussmaul's breathing** (air hunger): rapid deep breathing caused by stimulation of the respiratory centre by metabolic acidosis, e.g. in ketoacidosis
- **Cheyne–Stokes respiratory pattern**: apnoea/hyperpnoea; usually observed in the end stages of life; can also be associated with left ventricular failure (Trim, 2005)
- **hyperventilation**: usually anxiety related.

Adequacy of ventilation

Assess the adequacy of ventilation. Hypoxia/hypoxaemia can effect the:
- **heart rate**: initially tachycardia, can lead to bradycardia if severe
- **skin colour**: initially pallor; central cyanosis is a late sign (Smith, 2003), usually pre-terminal (in anaemia, severe hypoxaemia may not cause cyanosis and in chronic obstructive pulmonary disease (COPD) or congenital heart disease, cyanosis may be 'normal')
- **mental state**: agitation, drowsiness, confusion and impaired consciousness.

Other considerations

Other considerations when assessing breathing include:
- **casualty posture**: orthopnoea – assess the casualty's posture/position to determine whether it is conducive to maintaining a patent airway
- **tracheal position**: deviation of the trachea to one side indicates mediastinal shift, e.g. pneumothorax
- **chest percussion**: hyper-resonance suggests a pneumothorax while dullness suggests consolidation or presence of pleural fluid
- **emotional state**: a breathless casualty will be anxious
- **past medical history**: particularly respiratory related history and if the casualty has been prescribed respiratory related medications, e.g. inhalers, oxygen
- **respiratory related chest pain:** normally sharp, aggravated by deep breathing or coughing and localised to one particular area

- **cough**: common respiratory symptom, occurring when a deep inspiration is followed by an explosive expiration. The timing and duration of the cough is important:
  - cough that is worse at night: suggestive of asthma or heart failure
  - cough that is worse after eating: suggestive of oesophageal reflux
  - sudden cough: suggestive of foreign body
  - recent cough: suggestive of chest infection
  - chronic cough associated with a wheeze: suggestive of asthma
  - irritating chronic dry cough: suggestive of oesophageal reflux
  - chronic cough together with the production of large volumes of purulent sputum: suggestive of bronchiectasis
  - chronic cough which changes in character: suggestive of carcinoma of the lung
- **sputum**: if the casualty is expectorating sputum, note the colour and consistency:
  - white mucoid sputum: may be due to asthma or chronic bronchitis
  - purulent green or yellow sputum: due to a respiratory infection
  - blood-stained sputum: may be due to pulmonary embolism or carcinoma of the lung
  - frothy white or pink sputum: may be due to pulmonary oedema
  - thick, viscid sputum: may be due to severe asthma
  - thin, watery sputum: may be due to pulmonary oedema
  - foul-smelling sputum: may be due to respiratory tract infection
  - black specks: may be due to inhalation of smoke or coal dust
- **halitosis**: suggestive of poor oral hygiene or an upper respiratory tract infection
- **racial background or recent travel**: a casualty who has recently visited Asia may have been exposed to tuberculosis. Breathlessness following a long-haul flight could be a sign of pulmonary embolus.

Assessment of the circulation (and haemorrhage control)

Assessment of the circulation involves assessing the pulse, skin perfusion and cerebral perfusion.

Pulse

Assess the pulse. A normal resting pulse is 60–100 per minute. Abnormal findings include:

- **tachycardia** (heart rate >100): causes include anxiety, stress, pain, pyrexia, myocardial ischaemia, hypovolaemia and sympathetic stimulation
- **bradycardia** (heart rate <60): causes include ischaemic heart disease, medications, e.g. beta blockers, hypoxia/hypoxaemia and parasympathetic stimulation, e.g. during vomiting
- **rapid, weak and thready pulse**: characteristic of shock
- **full bounding or throbbing pulse**: causes include anaemia, heart block and heart failure; may also indicate sepsis
- **irregular pulse**: causes include cardiac arrhythmias, e.g. atrial fibrillation, and sometimes during inspiration/expiration.

Skin perfusion

Assess skin perfusion. Poor skin perfusion is usually characterised by cool peripheries, skin mottling, pallor, cyanosis and a delayed capillary refill (>2 seconds). Peripheral skin temperature is an important indicator when assessing the casualty. If the casualty is cool to the touch, this may indicate vasoconstriction and poor tissue perfusion; if the patient is hot to the touch, this may indicate vasodilation and possibly infection or even sepsis (Trim, 2005). To assess capillary refill:

1 explain the procedure to the casualty
2 blanch the sternum for five seconds, then release. A sluggish (delayed) capillary refill (>2 seconds) may be caused by circulatory shock, pyrexia or a cold ambient temperature (Jevon & Ewens, 2002).

Cerebral perfusion

Assess cerebral perfusion. Clinical signs of poor cerebral perfusion include deterioration in conscious level, confusion, agitation and lethargy.

Haemorrhage control

Control any external haemorrhage by applying direct pressure, using a sterile pad if possible.

Assessment of disability

Assessment of disability (casualty's neurological status) involves assessing level of consciousness using the 'AVPU' system and the pupils (size, equality and reaction to light). For completeness the Glasgow Coma Scale (GCS) is detailed in Appendix 2.1, though it is unlikely to be used in the first aid setting. In a casualty with known diabetes, an assessment of blood sugar may be helpful if a testing kit is at hand.

AVPU

The casualty's level of consciousness is the degree of awareness of the surrounding environment and arousal. It has two parts:
* arousal or wakefulness: being aware of the environment
* cognition: demonstrating an understanding of what the practitioner has said through an ability to perform tasks.

The casualty's conscious level can only be assessed by observing behaviour in response to different stimuli. This response to stimulation can be quantified and recorded by the simple neurological scoring system with the mnemonic AVPU:

- <u>A</u>lert

- Responsive to <u>V</u>erbal stimulation

- Responsive to <u>P</u>ainful stimulation

- <u>U</u>nresponsive (Jevon & Ewens, 2002).

Pupillary assessment

Pupillary assessment can be helpful. Altered pupil reaction, size or shape, together with other neurological signs, are a late sign of raised intracranial pressure. Before assessing the pupils note if there is any pre-existing irregularity with the pupils, e.g. cataracts, false eye or a previous eye injury.

Pupillary assessment should include the following:
- **size (mm)**: average size is 2–5 mm; both pupils should be equal in size. Factors that cause pupillary dilation include certain medications, e.g. tricyclics. Narcotics can cause pupillary constriction

- **shape**: should be round; abnormal shapes (oval or irregular) may indicate cerebral damage

- **reactivity to light**: a bright light source (usually from a pen torch) should be moved from the outer aspect of the eye towards the pupil – a brisk pupil constriction should follow. Following removal of the light source the pupil should return to its original size. The procedure should be repeated for the other eye. There should also be a consensual reaction to the light source, i.e. both eyes constrict when the light source is applied to the one. The reaction should be noted as brisk, sluggish or absent. NB A lens implant or a cataract can prevent the pupil from constricting to light

- **equality**: both pupils should be equal in shape and size and should react equally to light.

Blood sugar assessment

If would be helpful to assess the casualty's blood sugar. However, unless the casualty is a known diabetic and has a home blood sugar testing kit, it will not be possible to do this.

Exposure

Assess the casualty's temperature and establish whether the temperature is normal or if there is any hypothermia or pyrexia. To ensure adequate examination of the casualty, full exposure of the body may be necessary. The casualty's dignity must be respected and heat loss prevented.

Removing clothing

Removing the casualty's clothing can cause anxiety and feelings of vulnerability, as well as exposure to the elements. Therefore only remove clothing if it is absolutely essential. Some points to consider:

- obtain the casualty's consent where possible; explain why it is necessary to remove an item of clothing
- maintain the casualty's dignity
- if it is necessary to cut a garment, try to cut along the seams of trousers or sleeves
- if the casualty has a foot or leg injury, try to remove the shoe or boot before the ankle/leg becomes swollen
- if the casualty has sustained a possible spinal injury do not attempt to remove an upper garment
- if removing an upper garment when there is an upper limb injury, remove the uninjured arm before the injured arm; encourage the casualty to support the injured arm.

Removing a protective helmet

A protective helmet should only be removed if it is absolutely necessary, e.g. if it is impeding the casualty's breathing. If the casualty is breathing and has a patent airway leave the removal of a protective helmet to the emergency services (Keech, 2004). However, it may be necessary to proceed quickly, e.g. the casualty is unconscious with a compromised airway. In this situation try to find another person to help so that the neck can be supported and the head can be kept aligned with the spine during removal of the helmet.

Full-face helmet

While one person supports the casualty's neck and holds onto the lower jaw the second person should:

1 sit behind the casualty's head

2 undo or cut the straps of the helmet

3 place the fingers underneath the rim of the helmet

4 ease off the helmet – it may need to be tilted backwards to get it over the chin and then forwards to get it over the back of the head (St John Ambulance, 2002; Keech, 2004).

Open-face helmet

While one person supports the casualty's neck and holds onto the lower jaw the second person should:

1 sit behind the casualty's head

2 undo or cut the chin strap

3 place the fingers underneath the rim of the helmet

4 grip the sides of the helmet and pull them apart to take the pressure off the head

5 ease the helmet upwards and backwards off the casualty's head (St John Ambulance, 2002; Keech, 2004).

Do not remove the helmet unless it is absolutely necessary. Wait for the emergency services.

Secondary survey

Once it is established that the casualty is not in immediate danger, and no deficit is identified on primary survey, a secondary survey should be performed. Depending on the situation, this could involve:
- taking a history
- looking for external clues
- ascertaining the mechanics of injury
- assessing signs and symptoms
- undertaking a head to toe survey
  (St John Ambulance, 2002).

History

Take a history:
- casualty details, e.g. age, past medical history, contact address, next of kin, medications, etc.
- past medical history including any medications being taken
- details of injury/accident, e.g. time and how it happened, mechanics of injury (see below)
- when the casualty last had something to eat or drink.

As well as asking the casualty, also question bystanders, friends, work colleagues, relatives if appropriate.

External clues

Look for external clues, e.g. medications, MedicAlert® bracelet (Fig. 2.1). Observe the scene: is there anything suspicious?

Mechanics of injury

Information related to the mechanics of injury can be helpful because it can help predict the type and severity of injuries. Questions that could be asked include:

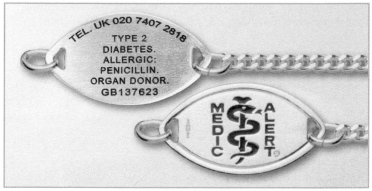

Figure 2.1 MedicAlert® bracelet. Reproduced with permission of MedicAlert®

- Was the casualty ejected out of the vehicle?
- Was the casualty wearing a seat belt?
- Was the casualty wearing a protective helmet?
- Did the casualty fall from a height? If so how did he land?
- In the case of a car crash, was the casualty's car hit on the side, from the front or from the back or did the car hit something else?
- Was the casualty a pedestrian? Did he hit the windscreen?

Signs and symptoms

Look for any signs and ask the casualty if there are any symptoms.

Head to toe survey

Undertake a head to toe survey (British Red Cross, 2003):

Head

Check for swelling, depressions, lacerations and bleeding; ensure to keep the head still and in alignment if a neck injury is suspected. Examine the nose and ears for blood and clear fluid – may indicate cerebral damage. Smell the casualty's breath for signs of alcohol, though never assume that a decrease in conscious level is due to alcohol.

Neck

Carefully check the back of the casualty's neck for swelling or tenderness; check for a medical ID tag. Ensure that the neck is kept still and in alignment if a neck injury is suspected. Loosen any tight clothing around the neck.

Chest

Check for chest movement and gently palpate to ascertain the presence of chest tenderness; look for wounds, bruising and swelling.

Abdomen

Gently palpate the casualty's abdomen to detect any evidence of bleeding and to identify any tenderness or rigidity in the abdomen; look for wounds, bruising and swelling.

Pelvis

Note any tenderness over the hips; check the clothing for signs of incontinence or bleeding from orifices.

Back

Ask the casualty if there is any back pain, numbness or tingling; if so, there may have been a back injury; therefore the casualty should not be moved.

Arms, hands, legs and ankles

Ask the casualty to raise each leg in turn and move each knee and ankle; look for any bleeding, bruising, deformity, tenderness or swelling; check the colour and temperature of the peripheries; check for a MedicAlert® bracelet (see Fig. 2.1).

Vital signs

Continually monitor the casualty's vital signs as appropriate.

Conclusion

Before undertaking an assessment of the casualty, the initial priority is to check for hazards. Once it is safe to approach, assess the casualty. Initially, a primary survey should be undertaken to assess for life-threatening conditions that require life-saving first aid. The comprehensiveness of the assessment required will depend on the situation. Once it is established that the casualty is not in immediate danger, a secondary survey can then be performed.

Appendix 2.1 The Glasgow Coma Scale

			Patient Name:					
			Hospital Number:					
			Ward:					
Date:			13	14	15	16		
Time:				30	30	30	30	
EYES OPEN C = eyes closed by swelling	Spontaneously	4						
	To speech	3						
	To pain	2						
	None	1						
BEST VERBAL RESPONSE T = ETT or Tracheostomy	Orientated	5						
	Confused	4						
	Inappropriate words	3						
	Incomprehensible sounds	2						
	None	1						
BEST MOTOR RESPONSE (Record best response) P = Paralysed	Obeys commands	6						
	Localises to pain	5						
	Flexes/withdraws to pain	4						
	Abnormal flexion	3						
	Extension	2						
	None	1						
TOTAL GLASGOW COMA SCORE			15	14	11	10	9	7	4	3
PUPILS + = Reacts − = No reaction S = Sluggish	RIGHT	Size						
		Reaction						
	LEFT	Size						
		Reaction						

LIMB MOVEMENTS Record Right (R) and Left (L) separately if there is a difference	A R M S	Normal Power	•	•					
		Mild weakness			L				
		Severe weakness				R	R		
		Abnormal flexion					R		
		Extension						•	
		No response							•
	L E G S	Normal Power	•	•					
		Mild weakness			L				
		Severe weakness				L	L	L	
		Extension						•	
		No response							•

PUPILS mm
1
2
3
4
5
6
7
8

Blood Pressure (mmHg)
240 220 210 200 190 180 170 160 150 140 130 120 110 100 90 80 70 60 50 40 30

Heart Rate (Beats/min)

TEMPERATURE °C

| Respiratory Rate | |
| Oxygen Saturation | |

Basic life support in adults

Introduction

Basic life support (BLS) refers to maintaining an open airway, supporting breathing and supporting circulation without the use of equipment other than a protective shield. BLS is often only a holding procedure, buying time while the means of reversing the underlying cause of the arrest can be obtained. In the community setting this is usually defibrillation.

The aim of this chapter is to understand the principles of basic life support in adults.

Chapter objectives
At the end of the chapter the reader will be able to:

- **Describe the initial assessment and sequence of actions in BLS**

- **Discuss the principles of chest compressions**

- **Outline the principles of opening the airway**

- **Discuss the principles of mouth-to-mouth ventilation**

- **Discuss the principles of mouth-to-nose and mouth-to-stoma ventilation**

- **Outline the principles of mouth-to-mask ventilation**

- **Describe a procedure for placing the casualty into a recovery position**

- **Describe the treatment for foreign body airway obstruction**

Initial assessment and sequence of actions in BLS

The initial assessment and sequence of actions in BLS are outlined in Figure 3.1, based on the Resuscitation Council (UK) algorithm for adult BLS (Resuscitation Council UK, 2005).

Check for dangers

The initial priority is always to check for dangers. Approach the casualty carefully, ensuring there is no danger either to the

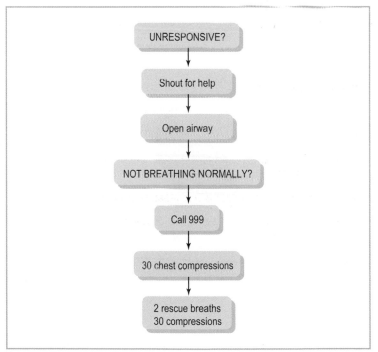

Figure 3.1 Resuscitation Council (UK) BLS algorithm. Reproduced with permission from the Resuscitation Council (UK)

rescuer or the casualty: look out for hazards, e.g. electricity, fire and traffic.

Check responsiveness

Gently shake the casualty's shoulders and ask loudly 'are you all right?' (Fig. 3.2).

Response: leave the casualty in the position found, provided there is no further danger. Establish the likely cause of the collapse (a more comprehensive casualty assessment is outlined in Chapter 2) and get help if necessary.

No response: shout out for help and open the airway.

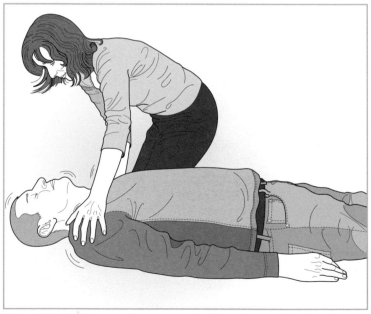

Figure 3.2 Check responsiveness: gently shake the casualty's shoulders and ask loudly, 'Are you alright?'

Open airway

Turn the casualty onto the back (unless full assessment is possible in the found position). Open the airway by tilting the head and lifting the chin (Fig. 3.3) (caution if cervical spine injury suspected – see below). Look in the mouth and remove any obvious obstruction and then assess for signs of normal breathing.

Assess for signs of normal breathing

While maintaining an open airway, assess for signs of normal breathing for no longer than 10 seconds: look for chest movement, listen at the casualty's mouth for breath sounds and feel for air on your cheek. During the first few minutes following a cardiac arrest,

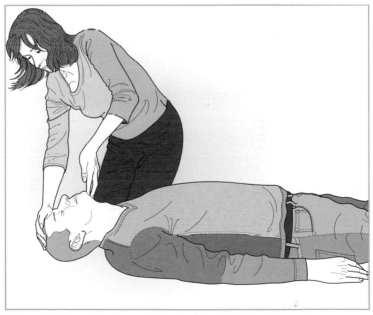

Figure 3.3 Open the airway: tilt the head and lift the chin

agonal gasps are often present – these should not be confused with normal breathing; in fact they are an indication to start CPR immediately (Resuscitation Council UK, 2005).

Checking for a carotid pulse can be difficult, is not included in the BLS guidelines and is not recommended for lay persons. Although in the hospital setting, nurses experienced in clinical assessment may prefer to also assess the carotid pulse for no longer than 10 seconds (often simultaneously with checking for signs of normal breathing) (Resuscitation Council UK, 2005), in the first aid setting this may not be easy. Assessing the casualty for signs of normal breathing as described above and not checking for a carotid pulse is recommended (Resuscitation Council UK, 2005).

Casualty breathing normally: place him in the recovery position, and ensure help is called

Casualty not breathing normally: send someone else to alert the emergency services (if alone, do this yourself) and then start CPR, chest compressions first. Recommended ratio of 30 compressions: 2 ventilations.

Principles of chest compressions

Chest compressions create blood flow by increasing intrathoracic pressure or directly compressing the heart. Even if chest compressions are being performed correctly, cardiac output is still only about 30% of normal with systolic blood pressures of between 60 and 80 mmHg being achieved. During chest compressions blood flow can be maximised by positioning the casualty horizontal, using the recommended chest compression force, duration, rate and ratio.

Duration

Cerebral and coronary perfusion is optimum when 50% of the cycle is devoted to chest compression phase and 50% to the chest relaxation phase.

Procedure

1 Ensure the casualty is supine, on a firm, flat surface
2 Kneel in the high kneeling position at the side of the casualty level with the chest, with the knees a shoulder-width apart
3 Place the heel of one hand in the centre of the casualty's chest
4 Position the heel of the other hand on top of the first hand
5 Interlock the fingers and lift them up to ensure that pressure is not exerted on the ribs, over the bottom end of the sternum or over the abdomen (Fig. 3.4)

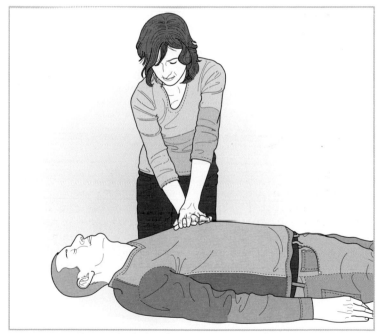

Figure 3.4 Chest compressions: leave the heel of one hand in the centre of the chest and place the heel of the other on top. Reproduced with permission from the Resuscitation Council (UK)

6 Position the shoulders vertically above the casualty, directly over your hands. Ensure the arms are straight and elbows are locked in position

7 Compress the chest vertically downwards approximately 4–5 cm (Fig. 3.5). It is important to release to allow ventricular filling. Compression/release times should be equal as this will help to maximise arterial pressures. Ensure the pressure is firm, controlled and not erratic. The force for compressions should come from flexing the hips. Lesser degrees of compression in smaller adults and greater degrees in larger adults may sometimes be required

8 Compress the chest at a rate of 100 per minute. A simple method of achieving the desired rate is to count out loud, '1-2-3-4-5', etc.

9 Leave the hands on the chest following each compression as your weight will control the rebound of the casualty's chest

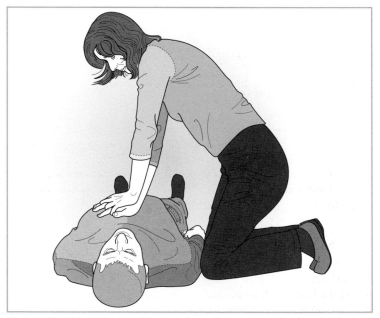

Figure 3.5 Chest compressions: apply vertical pressure down

10 Combine chest compressions with ventilations at a ratio of 30:2. If the paramedics intubate the casualty, compressions and ventilations can be asynchronous

Chest compression–only CPR

During the first few minutes following a cardiac arrest, which has not been caused by asphyxia, chest compressions only are just as effective as chest compressions and ventilations (Resuscitation Council UK, 2005). If unable or unwilling to perform mouth-to-mouth ventilation, rescuers are therefore encouraged to perform chest compressions only, even though chest compressions combined with ventilations is a significantly better method of CPR (Resuscitation Council UK, 2005). However, where a nurse would be expected to perform CPR on one of her patients, it is important that she ensures that she has access to an appropriate barrier device and is trained in its use.

Principles of opening the airway

Head tilt and chin lift

The head tilt/chin lift manoeuvre (see Fig. 3.3) is considered the most effective method of opening the airway of an unconscious casualty. In BLS it can achieve airway patency in 91% of cases. By stretching the anterior tissues of the neck, it displaces the tongue forward away from the posterior pharyngeal wall and lifts the epiglottis from the laryngeal opening.

Suspected cervical spine injury

If a cervical spine injury is suspected, lift the chin but try to avoid tilting the head. Causes of a cervical spine injury include head injury, road traffic accident, horse-riding accident, fall from a height, diving into shallow water and a rugby scrum accident.

Opening the airway is the first priority and a degree of head tilt may be unavoidable (Resuscitation Council UK and British Heart Foundation, 2003)

Jaw thrust

A jaw thrust (Fig. 3.6) is an alternative manoeuvre to open the airway and is particularly favoured if there is a suspected cervical spine injury (Committee on Trauma of the American College of Surgeons, 1997). However, a lone rescuer would find it very difficult to maintain a jaw thrust and perform BLS. In addition, it is a skill often only acquired by nurses working in such areas as A & E and Anaesthetics.

However, for completeness, a suggested method to perform a jaw thrust is:

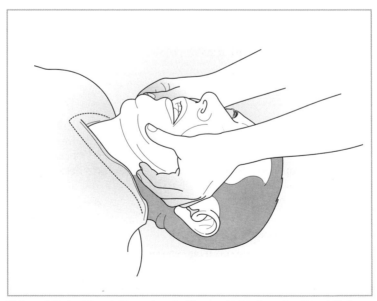

Figure 3.6 Jaw thrust. Reproduced with permission from the Resuscitation Council (UK)

- displace the mandible anteriorly (together with the tongue) using the index fingers positioned just proximal to the angles of the jaw
- apply pressure (at the same time) on the chin using the thumbs to help open the mouth.

Principles of mouth-to-mouth ventilation

Mouth-to-mouth ventilation is a quick, effective way to provide adequate oxygenation and ventilation in a casualty who is not breathing.

However, particular attention to the correct technique is essential. The most common cause of failure to ventilate is improper positioning of the head and chin.

Procedure

1 Position the casualty in a supine position

2 Kneel in a comfortable position with the knees a shoulder width apart, at the side of the casualty at the level of the nose and mouth (a wider base will be required to undertake compressions if only one person performing CPR)

3 Rest back to sit on the heels in the low kneeling position

4 If trained to do so, apply a face shield barrier device (Fig. 3.7)

5 Bend forwards from the hips leaning down towards the casualty's nose and mouth

6 While maintaining head tilt and chin lift, pinch the soft part of the casualty's nose using the index finger and thumb of the hand on the casualty's forehead

7 Open the casualty's mouth, maintain chin lift and take a breath in (Fig. 3.8)

8 Place your lips around the casualty's mouth ensuring a good seal

9 Blow steadily into the casualty's mouth over about 1 second watching for clear chest rise. Avoid high tidal volumes and the associated high

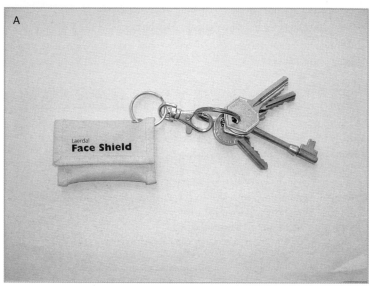

Figure 3.7 A Face shield barrier device

airway pressures as these may lead to gastric inflation and the
associated complications

10 While still maintaining head tilt and chin lift, remove your mouth and
watch for chest fall, as the air comes out

11 Repeat the procedure. If rescue breaths only are required, deliver
approximately 10 per minute

Ineffective delivery of breaths

If it is difficult to deliver effective breaths:
- ensure adequate head tilt and chin lift
- recheck the casualty's mouth and remove any obstruction
- ensure a good seal between your mouth and the casualty's mouth
- ensure the casualty's nose is pinched during ventilation.

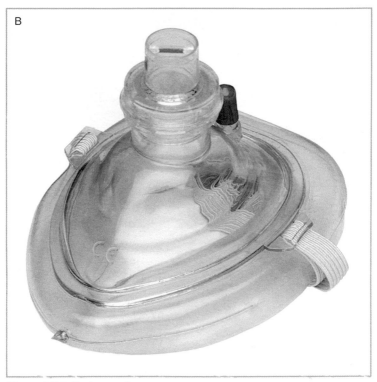

Figure 3.7 B Pocket mask

Do not attempt more than two breaths each time before re-starting chest compressions (Resuscitation Council UK, 2005).

Minimising gastric inflation

Gastric inflation is commonly associated with mouth-to-mouth ventilation. It occurs when the pressure in the oesophagus exceeds the opening pressure of the lower oesophageal sphincter pressure, resulting in the sphincter opening. During CPR the oesophageal sphincter relaxes, thus increasing the likelihood of gastric inflation.

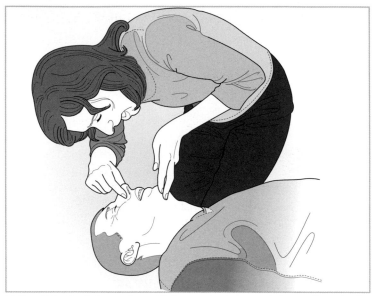

Figure 3.8 Mouth-to-mouth ventilation: open the casualty's mouth, maintain chin lift and take a breath in. Reproduced with permission from the Resuscitation Council (UK)

Complications of gastric inflation include:
- regurgitation
- aspiration
- pneumonia
- diaphragm elevation, restricted lung movements and reduced lung compliance.

To reduce the risk of gastric inflation it is important to deliver rescue breaths slowly over 2 seconds and at the lowest tidal volume (usually 700–1000 ml) to achieve clear visible chest rise. Although smaller tidal volumes would be safer, without supplementary oxygen they would provide inadequate oxygenation.

Principles of mouth-to-nose and mouth-to-stoma ventilation

There are some situations where mouth-to-nose ventilation may be preferred to mouth-to-mouth ventilation.

- Difficult mouth-to-mouth ventilation, e.g. if the casualty has unusual or absent dentition
- If there is an obstruction in the casualty's mouth that cannot be relieved
- While rescuing a casualty from water, when one hand is needed to support the body and therefore cannot be used to pinch the nose
- When resuscitation is being undertaken by a child (the mouth may not be large enough to ensure an adequate seal around an adult's mouth)
- For aesthetic reasons.

Procedure for mouth-to-nose ventilation

1. Release the casualty's nose and close the mouth
2. Sealing your mouth around the casualty's nose, blow in steadily as for the mouth-to-mouth technique (see above)
3. Open the casualty's mouth to let the breath out

Mouth-to-stoma ventilation

If the casualty has a stoma, e.g. following a laryngectomy, close off the mouth and nose with your thumb and fingers and then blow steadily into the stoma.

Principles of mouth-to-mask ventilation

Mouth-to-mask ventilation using a well-fitting pocket mask (Fig. 3.9) is an effective method of ventilation. Most pocket masks are transparent, thus enabling prompt detection of any vomit or blood in the airway. A one-way valve directs the casualty's expired air away from the rescuer.

Method

1 Position yourself behind the patient's head
2 Ensure the casualty is supine and tilt the head back
3 Apply the mask to the face, pressing down with the thumbs (Fig. 3.9)
4 Lift the chin into the mask by applying pressure behind the angles of the jaw
5 Ventilate the patient with sufficient air to cause visible chest rise. Observe for chest rise and fall
6 Adopt a comfortable position for ventilation and avoid static postures

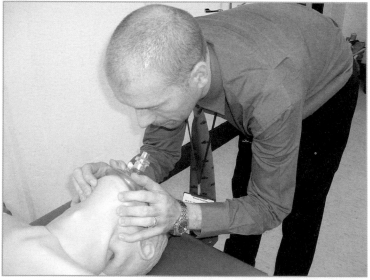

Figure 3.9 Mouth-to-mask ventilation: apply the mask to the face, pressing down with the thumbs

For single rescuer CPR, it is usually better to adopt a position to the side of the patient's head to facilitate the switching between ventilations and chest compressions.

Procedure for placing the casualty into a recovery position

Although there are a number of recovery positions currently advocated, no single one can be endorsed. However, the position adopted should:
- be stable
- maintain a patent airway
- maintain a stable cervical spine
- avoid application of pressure on the chest that restricts breathing
- minimise the risk of aspiration
- limit pressure on bony prominences and peripheral nerves
- enable visualisation of the casualty's breathing and colour
- allow access to the casualty for interventions
- be easy and safe to achieve (including repositioning if required).

The Resuscitation Council UK (2005) suggests the following technique for placing an adult into the recovery position (see Fig. 3.13):
1 remove the casualty's spectacles
2 kneel beside the casualty and ensure that both the legs are straight
3 place the casualty's arm which is nearest to you out at right angles to the body, elbow bent with the hand palm facing upwards (Fig. 3.10)
4 bringing the casualty's far arm across the chest, hold the back of the hand against the casualty's cheek which is nearest to you (Fig. 3.11)
5 using the other hand, grasp the casualty's far leg just above the knee and pull it up, keeping the foot on the ground
6 while keeping the casualty's hand pressed against the cheek, pull on the leg to roll the casualty towards you onto the side (Fig. 3.12)
7 adjust the casualty's upper leg, ensuring that both the hip and knee are bent at right angles (Fig. 3.13)

8 tilt the casualty's head back to ensure that the airway remains patent

9 if necessary, adjust the hand under the cheek to help ensure the head remains tilted

10 monitor the casualty's vital signs

11 monitor the peripheral circulation in the lower arm; pressure on this area should be kept to a minimum. Turn the casualty to the opposite side if the recovery position has been maintained for more than 30 minutes.

Treatment for foreign body airway obstruction

Complete obstruction of the airway by a foreign body is a life-threatening emergency and recognition is the key to a successful outcome (Resuscitation Council UK, 2005). It is often

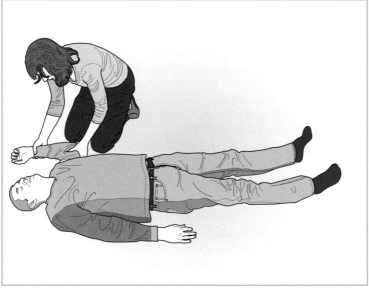

Figure 3.10 Recovery position: place the casualty's arm at right angles to the body, elbow bent with the hand palm facing upwards

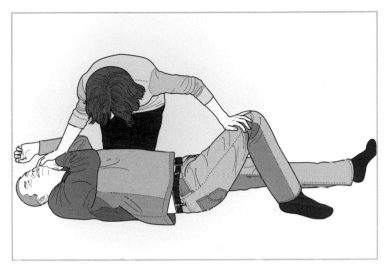

Figure 3.11 Recovery position: bringing the casualty's far arm across the chest, hold the back of the hand against the casualty's cheek

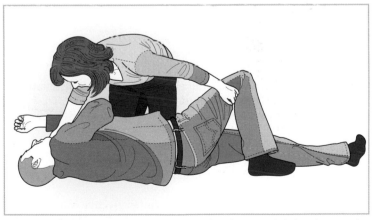

Figure 3.12 Recovery position: while keeping the casualty's hand pressed against the cheek, pull on the leg to roll the casualty onto the side

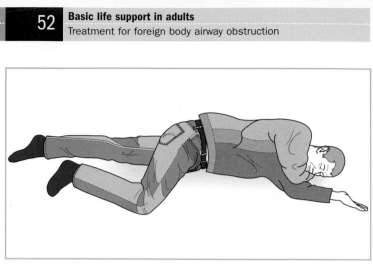

Figure 3.13 The recovery position

characterised by a sudden inability to talk, maximal respiratory effort, development of cyanosis and clutching of the neck. In partial airway obstruction, the casualty will be distressed, may cough and may have a wheeze. In complete airway obstruction, the casualty will be unable to speak, breathe or cough and will eventually collapse and become unconscious.

Treatment

The treatment algorithm for adult choking based on Resuscitation Council (UK) guidelines (2005) is depicted in Figure 3.14. The Resuscitation Council (UK) recommends the following sequence of actions:

Mild airway obstruction (casualty has an effective cough):
• Just encourage the casualty to continue coughing

Severe airway obstruction (casualty has an ineffective cough, but is conscious):
• Stand to the side and just behind the casualty
• Support the casualty's chest with one hand and lean him well forward

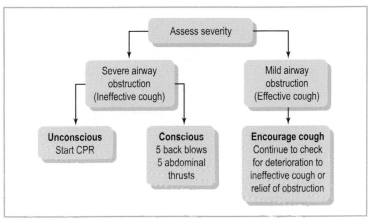

Figure 3.14 Resuscitation Council (UK) adult choking treatment algorithm. Reproduced with permission from the Resuscitation Council (UK)

- Deliver up to five back blows between the scapulae using the heel of the other hand (Fig. 3.15), checking after each one to see if it has dislodged the foreign body. If five back blows are unsuccessful, proceed to abdominal thrusts
- Stand behind the casualty, place both arms around his upper abdomen and lean him forward
- Position a clenched fist between the casualty's umbilicus and bottom end of the sternum
- Clasp the fist with the other hand and pull sharply inwards and upwards, applying up to five thrusts (Fig. 3.16)
- If abdominal thrusts are also unsuccessful, continue alternating five back blows and five abdominal thrusts

Severe airway obstruction (casualty unconscious). If the casualty loses consciousness:
- Help the casualty to the floor
- Ensure the emergency services have been alerted (if not already)
- Start CPR following the BLS guidelines described earlier in this chapter, i.e. 30 compressions: 2 ventilations (even if the casualty has a palpable pulse)

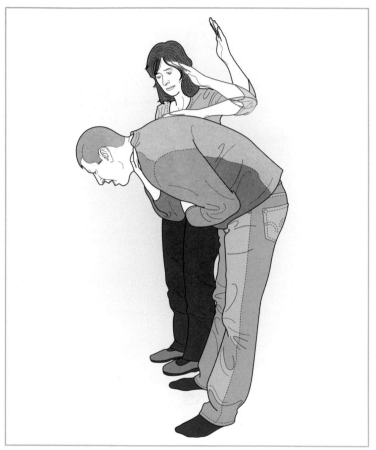

Figure 3.15 Choking casualty: deliver up to five sharp slaps between the scapulae using the heel of the hand

Successful treatment

If treatment is successful, but the casualty has a persistent cough, dysphagia or still has 'something stuck in his throat' or abdominal thrusts were required, advise him to seek medical help.

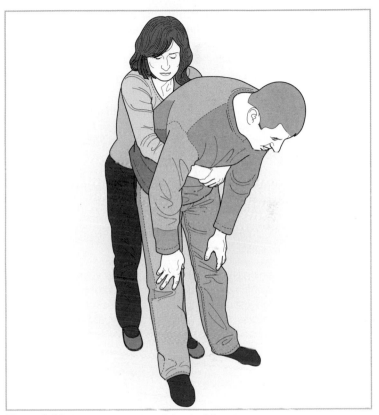

Figure 3.16 Choking casualty: abdominal thrusts

Adult guidelines for use in children

Children often do not receive CPR because potential rescuers are concerned that they may cause harm; this fear is unfounded and it is far better to adopt the adult sequence for BLS than do nothing (Resuscitation Council UK, 2006a). Historically paediatric CPR has not been taught on adult CPR sessions and only nurses with a duty to respond to paediatric emergencies are taught paediatric CPR.

However, those taught adult BLS, but who have no specific knowledge of paediatric resuscitation, should use the adult sequence; with, ideally, some modifications:

• Deliver five initial ventilations before starting chest compressions

• If alone, perform CPR first for 1 minute, then alert the emergency services

• Compress the chest approximately 1/3 of the depth using two fingers in an infant (< 1 year of age) and 1–2 hands in a child (> 1 year of age) as required to achieve adequate depth of compression (Resuscitation Council (UK), 2005).

In addition, the guidelines for relief of foreign body airway obstruction in adults can be implemented in children > 1 year of age.

Conclusion

BLS refers to maintaining an open airway, supporting breathing and supporting circulation without the use of equipment other than a protective shield. Often just a holding procedure, effective BLS buys time while the means of reversing the underlying cause of the arrest (usually defibrillation) can be obtained. This chapter has provided an overview to BLS in adults.

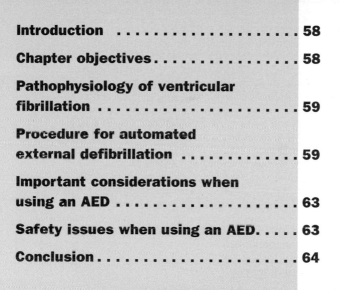

Automated external defibrillation

Automated external defibrillation

Introduction

Over 270 000 people in the UK suffer a myocardial infarction each year and about 30% die before reaching hospital due to cardiac arrest (British Heart Foundation, 2005). Most cardiac arrests occurring in the out-of-hospital setting are caused by ventricular fibrillation/pulseless ventricular tachycardia, the definitive treatment for which is early defibrillation.

Defibrillation is the delivery of an electrical current to the myocardium to terminate ventricular fibrillation (VF). Modern automated external defibrillators (AEDs) can be used by a wide range of personnel, both professional and non-professional, as audible and/or visual prompts guide the user through the procedure. The widespread deployment of AEDS in public places in the community enables early defibrillation.

The aim of this chapter is to understand the principles of automated external defibrillation.

Chapter objectives
At the end of the chapter the reader will be able to:

- Discuss the pathophysiology of ventricular fibrillation

- Outline the procedure for automated external defibrillation

- List the important considerations when using an AED

- Discuss the safety issues when using an AED

Pathophysiology of ventricular fibrillation

Ventricular fibrillation (VF) (Fig. 4.1) is the commonest primary arrhythmia at the onset of a cardiac arrest in adults. In the community approximately 80–90% of cardiac arrests in adults are caused by VF.

VF is an eminently treatable rhythm with most eventual survivors of a cardiac arrest coming from this group. Early defibrillation is the definitive treatment; the chances of success decline substantially with each minute's delay to defibrillation. There is a lower decline if there is adequate BLS. The widespread deployment of AEDs (Fig. 4.2) enables early defibrillation, before the arrival of the emergency services.

Procedure for automated external defibrillation

The following procedure for automated external defibrillation is based on the Resuscitation Council (UK) guidelines for automated external defibrillation (Fig. 4.3) (Resuscitation Council UK, 2005) (although some older AEDs may not be or can't be re-programmed to reflect the 2005 guidelines, still use them and follow the voice / visual prompts, even though they are configured to the Resuscitation Council UK 2000 guidelines (Resuscitation Council UK, 2006).

1 Confirm cardiac arrest following the BLS guidelines described in Chapter 3 and ensure the emergency services are alerted

2 Switch on AED and follow spoken and/or visual prompts. If possible ask someone else to continue CPR

3 Prepare the casualty's skin as necessary; ensure that the skin is dry and quickly remove any excess hair. This will help ensure good contact

PIN 804700

Figure 4.1 Ventricular fibrillation. Reproduced with permission from Jevon P (2002) **Advanced cardiac life support**. Elsevier, Edinburgh

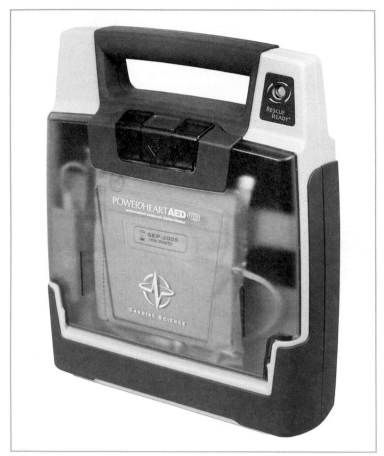

Figure 4.2 An AED. Reproduced with permission from Cardiac Science Holdings (UK) Limited

4 Attach the defibrillation electrodes following manufacturer's recommendations; one to the right of the sternum below the right clavicle and one vertically in the mid-axillary line level with the V6 ECG electrode position or the female breast (Fig. 4.4)

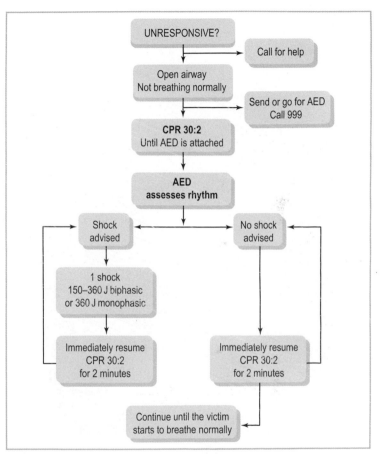

Figure 4.3 Resuscitation Council UK algorithm for automated defibrillation. Reproduced with permission from the Resuscitation Council (UK)

5 Ensure nobody is touching the casualty during ECG analysis by the AED. This is to prevent artefactual errors during ECG analysis

6 If shock is advised, shout 'stand clear' and perform a visual check to ensure all personnel are clear

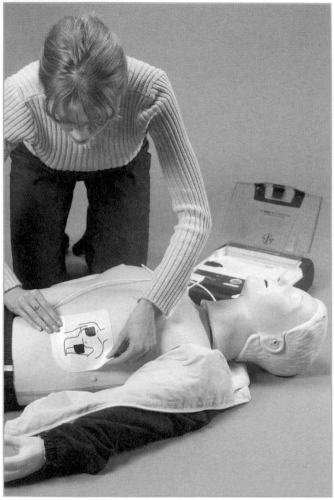

Figure 4.4 Automated external defibrillation. Attach the defibrillation electrodes, following manufacturer's recommendations: one to the right of the sternum below the right clavicle and one over the cardiac apex. Reproduced with permission from RTO, Learning Centre, Walsall Hospitals NHS Trust

7 After ensuring all personnel are clear of the casualty, press the shock button as indicated

8 Continue as advised by the voice/visual prompts

9 If no shock is advised, resume CPR, 30 compressions: 2 ventilations and continue as advised by voice/visual prompts

Important considerations when using an AED

• Safety precautions should be observed (see below)

• Ensure the emergency services are alerted first before using an AED

• CPR should be started if an AED is not immediately available

• If more than one rescuer is present, one can continue CPR while the other prepares the AED

• Some AEDs require the operator to press an 'analyse' button, while others automatically begin analysis once the electrodes are attached to the casualty's chest

• If the casualty has a hairy chest, the defibrillation electrodes may stick to the hairs, resulting in high transthoracic impedance – hence the importance of shaving the chest prior to electrode application. Do not delay AED use if razor not at hand

• Standard AEDs are currently not suitable for paediatric use (<8 years of age); however, some do have a paediatric lead attachment

• Some AEDs are fully automatic, i.e. if a shockable rhythm is recognised it will automatically charge up and defibrillate the casualty without the need for the operator to press a 'shock' button

Safety issues when using an AED

There are a number of safety issues when using an AED. It is important to:

• confirm cardiac arrest before applying the AED

• remove GTN patches as they pose an explosion hazard

- avoid direct and indirect contact with the casualty. All personnel should be well away from the bed and not touching the casualty. Be wary of wet surroundings

- remove oxygen away from the casualty

- shout 'stand clear' and check all personnel are safely clear prior to defibrillation

- place the defibrillation electrodes 12–15 cm away from an implanted pacing unit (most units are below the left clavicle, therefore the standard positioning of electrodes can be adopted).

Conclusion

Most cardiac arrests occurring in the community are caused by ventricular fibrillation/pulseless ventricular tachycardia, the definitive treatment for which is early defibrillation. This chapter has provided an overview of automated external defibrillation. The safety considerations have been highlighted.

Recognising respiratory failure and shock in infants and children

CHAPTER

5

Recognising respiratory failure and shock in infants and children

Introduction

Cardiopulmonary arrests in children are rarely sudden events and generally follow a period of profound hypoxia associated with respiratory failure and/or shock. As a result, by the time the child has deteriorated into a state of cardiopulmonary arrest, all the organs of the body will have suffered from the effects of hypoxia and ischaemia.

The prompt recognition and effective treatment of potential respiratory failure and shock in children is therefore essential if the dire situation of cardiopulmonary arrest and its associated poor prognosis is to be avoided.

It is therefore essential to be able to recognise that the child is ill and to alert the emergency services. The rapid assessment of the respiratory, cardiovascular and neurological functions, together with an assessment of the child's general appearance, can help to ascertain whether the child is seriously ill or not.

The aim of this chapter is to understand a systematic approach to recognising respiratory failure and shock in infants and children.

Chapter objectives
At the end of the chapter the reader will be able to:

- **Discuss the assessment of respiratory function**

- **Outline the assessment of cardiovascular function**

- **Describe the assessment of neurological function**

- **Discuss the assessment of the child's general appearance**

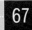
Assessment of respiratory function

The rapid assessment of respiratory function involves the evaluation of:

- work of breathing
- effectiveness of breathing
- adequacy of ventilation.

Work of breathing

Healthy spontaneous breathing is quiet and is accomplished with minimal effort. An increased respiratory rate, chest recession, noisy respirations, accessory muscle use and nasal flaring are signs of an increased work of breathing.

Respiratory rate

- Normal respiratory rates are detailed in Table 5.1
- Tachypnoea at rest can be caused by airway disease, lung disease or metabolic acidosis
- Tachypnoea is usually one of the first indications of respiratory distress
- Slow or irregular respirations in acutely ill infants and children is an ominous sign. Possible causes include fatigue, hypothermia and CNS

Table 5.1 Normal respiratory rates by age at rest (reproduced from ALSG, with kind permission)

Age (years)	Respiratory rate (breaths per minute)
<1	30–40
1–2	25–35
2–5	25–30
5–12	20–25
>12	15–20

depression. A slow respiratory rate in an exhausted child is a sign of deterioration, rather than improvement, and is a pre-terminal sign

- A trend of respiratory rates can be very useful and is sometimes more accurate than the first recorded rate (American Academy of Pediatrics, 2000)

Chest recession

- Intercostal, subcostal or sternal recession are signs of increased work of breathing (Fig. 5.1)
- Particularly visible in infants because their chest walls are more compliant – the chest wall is less muscular and thinner and the inward excursion between the ribs of the skin and soft tissue is more visible (American Academy of Pediatrics, 2000)
- If seen in older children (i.e. over 6 years of age) probably indicative of serious respiratory difficulties
- Degree of recession correlates with severity of respiratory distress

Noisy respirations

- Stridor: an inspiratory, high-pitched sound indicating partial upper airway obstruction; causes include croup, foreign body aspiration, infection and oedema
- Wheeze: whistling sound more pronounced on expiration indicating narrowing of the lower airways; two most common causes are asthma (generally in >1 year) and bronchiolitis (generally in <1 year)
- Grunting: short low-pitched sound resulting from exhalation against a partially closed glottis; it is an attempt to keep the alveoli open for gas exchange (and prevent airway collapse at the end of expiration); a sign of serious respiratory distress and is characteristically observed in infants

Accessory muscle use

- Use of the sternomastoid muscle may result in bobbing of the head up and down with each breath – on inhalation the neck is extended and on exhalation the head falls forward resulting in the characteristic 'head bobbing' effect

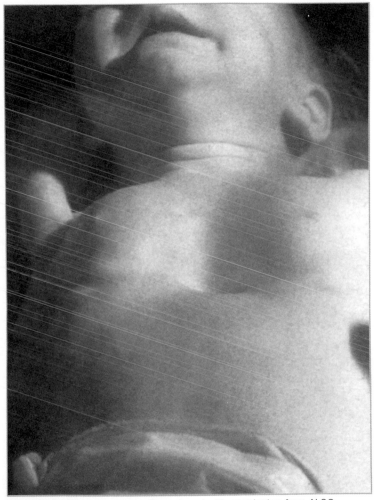

Figure 5.1 Chest recession. Reproduced with permission from ALSG

Nasal flaring

- Nasal flaring (exaggerated opening of the nostrils) is commonly seen in infants with respiratory distress

Child position

- Sniffing position: the child is making an attempt to line up the axes of the airways to open the airway and maximise airflow
- Tripod position: leaning forward on outstretched arms in an attempt to use accessory muscles

A child with depressed cerebral function, e.g. due to poisoning or a raised intracranial pressure, may present with respiratory inadequacy without the signs of increased work of breathing. This is due to a depressed respiratory drive.

Effectiveness of breathing

The effectiveness of breathing can be assessed by:
- chest movement
- air entry: look, listen and feel for signs of breathing.

Signs of inadequate ventilation

The assessment of heart rate, skin colour and mental status can help to determine whether ventilation is adequate.

Heart rate

- Initially tachycardia in the older infant and child (a non-specific sign)
- Severe hypoxia leads to bradycardia (a pre-terminal sign)

Skin colour

- Initially pallor. Hypoxia will lead to catecholamine release, causing vasoconstriction of the skin
- Central cyanosis is a late and pre-terminal sign of hypoxia

- If the child is anaemic, cyanosis may not be present even when hypoxia is severe

- Cyanosis may be 'normal' if the child has congenital heart disease

- In dark-skinned children, the lips and mucous membranes may be the best places to observe skin colour (American Academy of Pediatrics, 2000)

Mental status

Hypoxia will affect the mental status of the child. Initially, the child may be agitated, drowsy, or may fail to recognise/acknowledge the parents. If uncorrected this may lead to unconsciousness and generalised muscular hypotonia (floppy child). A useful method of rapidly assessing the mental status is by using the AVPU scale:

- Alert

- Responds to voice

- Responds to painful stimuli

- Unconscious

AVPU categorises motor response based on simple responses to stimuli (American Academy of Pediatrics, 2000).

Assessment of cardiovascular function

Assessment of cardiovascular function includes evaluation of:
- heart rate
- pulse volume
- capillary refill
- skin temperature
- respiratory system
- mental status.

Heart rate

- Normal heart rates are shown in Table 5.2

- Tachycardia is a non-specific sign (numerous causes of tachycardia including anxiety, excitement, pyrexia and pain)

Table 5.2 Normal range of heart rates by age (reproduced from ALSG, with kind permission)

Age (years)	Heart rate (beats per minute)
<1	110–160
1–2	100–150
2–5	95–140
5–12	80–120
>12	60–100

- Initially an increase in heart
- Bradycardia is an ominous sign
- A trend of increasing or decreasing heart rate recordings may be useful, suggesting worsening hypoxia or shock or improvement following effective treatment (American Academy of Pediatrics, 2000)

Pulse volume

- Absent peripheral pulses and weak central pulses indicate poor cardiac output and are signs of advanced stages of shock

Capillary refill

- The technique for measuring capillary refill is discussed on page 24. Although using a digit or foot (Fig. 5.2) has been common practice, as in adults, the sternum or forehead are more frequently used. The normal capillary refill is up to two seconds, as long as the child is not in a cold environment

Skin temperature

- If perfusion is adequate the child's skin near the wrists and ankles should be warm
- When cardiac output decreases cooling of the skin starts peripherally and extends proximally towards the trunk
- As shock worsens, a line of coldness can be identified moving centrally
- If the child is cold, core perfusion may be normal despite 'abnormal' skin perfusion due to peripheral shutdown

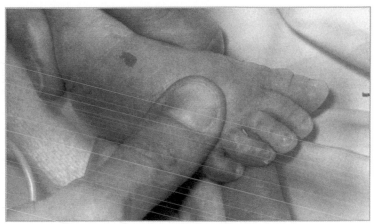

Figure 5.2 Capillary refill. Reproduced with permission from ALSG

Respiratory system

- Metabolic acidosis resulting from circulatory failure will cause tachypnoea and an increased depth of respiration (without chest recession)

Mental status

- Poor cerebral perfusion will cause agitation, drowsiness and then unconsciousness

Assessment of neurological function

A rapid assessment of neurological function involves evaluating conscious level, posture and pupils:

- Conscious level: use the AVPU scale (see p. 71); applying pressure to the sternum or pulling frontal hair are two acceptable methods of delivering the painful central stimulus (ALSG, 2005); a child who only responds to pain has a significant degree of coma corresponding to 8 or less on the Glasgow Coma Scale (ALSG, 2005)

- Pupils: causes of an abnormal pupillary response include drugs, hypoxia, convulsions and impending brain stem herniation; dilatation, unreactivity or inequality indicate a possible serious cerebral disorder (ALSG, 2001).

Neurological function can be adversely affected by both respiratory and cardiovascular dysfunction. In addition, neurological dysfunction can adversely affect both of these systems.

Assessment of the child's general appearance

The child's general appearance provides an indication to the adequacy of ventilation, oxygenation, tissue perfusion, cerebral perfusion and neurological function. A rapid assessment of the child's general appearance is therefore helpful when ascertaining how severe the illness or injury is, the need for treatment and the response to therapy.

The so-called 'tickles' (TICLS) mnemonic (American Academy of Pediatrics, 2000) can help with the assessment of the child's general appearance:

- Tone: good muscle tone or limp, listless or flaccid? Is the child vigorous and resisting examination?
- Interactiveness: how alert is the child? Attentive and easily distracted? Reaching for, grasping and playing with a toy? Uninterested in playing or interacting?
- Consolability: consoled or comforted by the carer? Crying and agitation unrelieved by gentle reassurance?
- Look/gaze: good eye contact? 'Nobody home', glassy-eyed stare?
- Speech/cry: speech or cry, strong and spontaneous or weak, muffled or hoarse?

An alert, interactive child may still be critically ill, e.g. in a toxicological or trauma emergency.

Conclusion

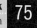

Cardiopulmonary arrests in children are rarely sudden events and generally follow a period of profound hypoxia associated with respiratory failure and/or shock. It is therefore essential to be able to recognise that the child is ill and to alert the emergency services. In this chapter a rapid assessment of the respiratory, cardiovascular and neurological functions, together with an assessment of the child's general appearance has been described.

Basic life support in infants and children

Introduction

The aetiology of cardiopulmonary arrests in infants and children differs to that in adults. They are normally secondary to either respiratory or circulatory failure, and rarely result from a primary cardiac event. Respiratory failure is the most common cause.

Historically, paediatric CPR has not been taught on adult CPR sessions and only nurses with a duty to respond to paediatric emergencies are taught paediatric CPR. Children often do not receive CPR because potential rescuers are concerned that they may cause harm; this fear is unfounded and it is far better to adopt the adult sequence fo BLS (Chapter 3) than do nothing (Resuscitation Council UK, 2006a). Rescuers who have been taught adult BLS, but have no specific knowledge on paediatric resuscitation, should use the adult sequence; with, ideally, some modifications:

- Deliver 5 initial ventilations before starting chest compressions
- If alone, perform CPR first for 1 minute, then alert the emergency services
- Compress the chest approximately 1/3 of the depth using 2 fingers in an infant (< 1 year of age) and 1–2 hands in a child (> 1 year of age) as required to achieve adequate depth of compression (Resuscitation Council UK, 2005)

In addition, the guidelines for relief of foreign body airway obstruction in adults described in Chapter 3 can be implemented in children > 1 year of age.

Training in paediatric BLS is recommended for healthcare professionals who have a duty to respond to paediatric emergencies, who are working in teams and who are in a position to receive enhanced training (Resuscitation Council UK, 2006a). However, it is acknowledged that some readers this book have a particular interest in paediatric BLS, nce this chapter.

The aim of this chapter is to understand the principles of S in infants and children.

Chapter objectives
At the end of the chapter the reader will be able to:

- Discuss the initial assessment and sequence of actions in BLS

- Outline the principles of basic airway management

- Describe the principles of mouth-to-mouth ventilation

- Discuss the principles of chest compressions

- Describe the recovery position

- Outline the management of foreign body airway obstruction

Age definitions for BLS in infants and children

Infant <1 year
Child between 1 year and puberty

Initial assessment and sequence of actions in BLS

The initial assessment and sequence of actions in paediatric BLS are outlined in the Resuscitation Council UK paediatric BLS algorithm (Fig. 6.1). On finding a collapsed, apparently lifeless infant/child, ensure it is safe to approach and then check responsiveness.

Check responsiveness

Infant: gently rub the chest, blow on the face, tickle the feet.

Child: gently stimulate the child. Do not shake the child if he has a suspected cervical spinal injury

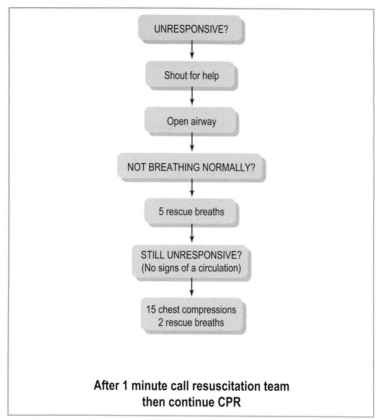

Figure 6.1 Resuscitation Council (UK) Paediatric BLS algorithm (health care professionals with a duty to respond). Reproduced with permission from the Resuscitation Council (UK)

Response: leave the infant/child in the position found, provided there is no further danger. Establish the likely cause of the collapse and get help if necessary.

No response: call out for help and proceed to assessing the airway. If there is no history of trauma, consider moving the infant/small child near to a phone so that the emergency services can be quickly alerted.

Open airway

Turn the infant/child onto the back (unless full assessment is possible in the position found). Open the airway by tilting the head and lifting the chin (neutral position in an infant). Look in the mouth and remove any obvious obstruction and then check breathing. If the child has a suspected cervical spine injury, try to open the airway using the jaw thrust technique (see Chapter 3); if this is unsuccessful, apply head tilt a small amount at a time until the airway is open (Resuscitation Council UK, 2005).

Check breathing

While maintaining an open airway check for signs of breathing (more than an occasional gasp or weak attempts at breathing) for up to 10 seconds:
• Look for chest movement
• Listen for airflow at the mouth and nose
• Feel for airflow on your cheek.

It can sometimes be difficult to establish whether the infant/child is breathing and it is important to differentiate ineffective, gasping or obstructed respirations from effective respirations. If uncertain whether the infant/child is breathing deliver rescue breaths.

Infant/child breathing normally: place in the recovery position (caution if history of trauma), check for continued breathing and ensure help is on the way.

Infant/child not breathing normally or is making agonal gasps: send someone else for help and deliver rescue breaths.

Breath

Deliver five initial breaths observing for any gag or cough response.

Assess signs of circulation

Allow up to 10 seconds to assess for signs of circulation: look, listen and feel for signs of breathing, coughing or movement of the infant/child. Also check for the pulse (if trained to do so) for no longer than 10 seconds:

Infant: check for the brachial pulse – short, chubby necks in infants makes checking for the carotid pulse difficult. The brachial pulse is located on the inside of the infant's upper arm, in between the elbow and the shoulder (Fig. 6.2).

Child: check for the carotid pulse (Fig. 6.3) – locate the thyroid cartilage (Adam's apple) with two or three fingers from one hand (maintain head tilt with the other), slide the fingers into the groove in between the trachea and sternocleidomastoid muscles and then gently palpate.

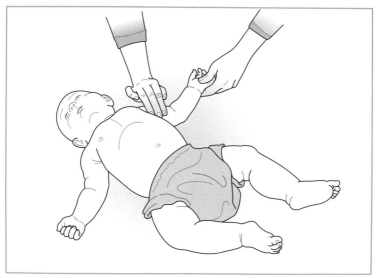

Figure 6.2 Checking for a brachial pulse in an infant

Only check the pulse if trained to do so, as it can be difficult reliably to determine its presence or absence. Teaching lay persons how to check for the pulse is not recommended. Instead they should be taught to look for signs of circulation in response to rescue breaths.

Signs of circulation: continue rescue breaths at a rate of 20 per minute and check for signs of circulation every minute.

No signs of circulation or unsure or pulse < 60 with poor perfusion: compress the chest at a rate of 100 per minute combining the compressions with rescue breaths at a ratio of 15:2 (15 compressions to 2 rescue breaths).

When to get help

More than one rescuer: one starts BLS while the other alerts the emergency services.

Lone rescuer: perform BLS for one minute before alerting the emergency services (it may be possible to carry an infant/small

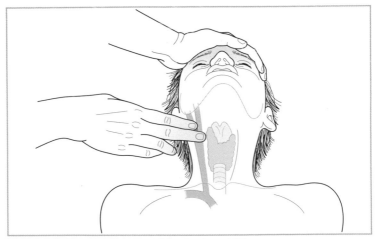

Figure 6.3 Checking for a carotid pulse in a child

child and perform CPR and get help simultaneously). In a witnessed, sudden collapse, the cause is likely to be a cardiac problem – alert the emergency services first (defibrillation may be required), then start CPR.

Principles of basic airway management

The airway in an unconscious child can easily become obstructed by a combination of flexion of the neck, relaxation of the jaw, displacement of the tongue against the posterior wall of the pharynx and collapse of the hypopharynx. In some cases just opening the airway may revive the child.

The airway can be opened by tilting the head and lifting the chin (Fig. 6.4). This will help to open the airway and bring the tongue forward from the posterior wall of the pharynx (the tongue is the most common cause of airway obstruction in an unconscious child). The neutral position in an infant and the sniffing the morning air position in a child are recommended.

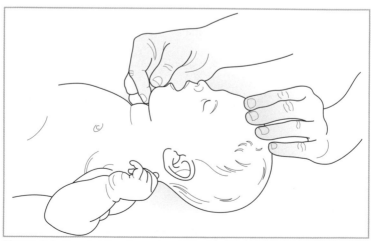

Figure 6.4 Opening the airway: head tilt, chin lift

Care should be taken not to press on the soft tissues under the chin as this may obstruct the airway. Blind finger sweeps are not recommended (ERC, 1998). Although cervical spine injuries are rare in infants and children, if there is a history of trauma, the jaw thrust rather than head tilt/chin lift is preferred.

Principles of mouth-to-mouth ventilation

Mouth-to-mouth ventilation is a quick, effective way to provide adequate oxygenation and ventilation in a casualty who is not breathing.

However, particular attention to the correct technique is essential. The most common cause of failure to ventilate is improper positioning of the head and chin.

Mouth-to-mouth and nose ventilation (infant)

1 Position the infant in a supine position (preferably on a table or similar)
2 Place the infant's head in a neutral position and maintain head tilt and chin lift
3 If trained to do so, apply a face shield barrier device
4 Take a deep breath in
5 Bend forwards from the hips leaning down towards the infant's nose and mouth (Fig. 6.5)
6 Place your lips around the infant's lips and nose, and ensure an airtight seal
7 Breathe out steadily into the infant's mouth and nose over 1–1.5 seconds and observe for chest rise. The correct breath volume is one that causes the chest to rise, without causing excessive gastric distension
8 While still maintaining a neutral position and chin lift, remove your mouth and watch for chest fall, as the air comes out

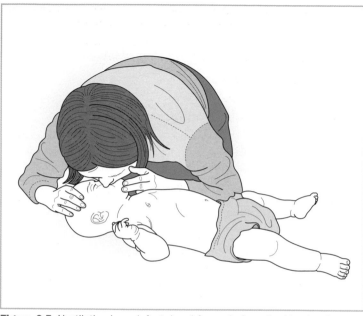

Figure 6.5 Ventilation in an infant: bend forwards from the hips leaning down towards the infant's nose and mouth

9 Take another breath in (pausing to take a breath will maximise the oxygen content and minimise the carbon dioxide content in the delivered breaths and repeat steps 5–9

10 Deliver five initial breaths in total

If the rescuer has a small mouth it may not be possible to cover both the infant's nose and mouth. In this situation mouth-to-nose ventilation may be adequate.

Mouth-to-mouth ventilation (child)

1 Position the child in a supine position (a smaller child preferably on a table or similar)

2 Kneel in a comfortable position with the knees a shoulder-width apart, at the side of the child at the level of the nose and mouth

3 Rest back to sit on the heels in the low kneeling position

4 If trained to do so, apply a face shield barrier device

5 Ensure head tilt and chin lift

6 Pinch the soft part of the child's nose

7 Take a deep breath in

8 Bend forwards from the hips leaning down towards the child's nose and mouth

9 Place your lips around the child's lips and ensure an airtight seal

10 Breathe out steadily into the child's mouth over 1–1.5 seconds and observe for chest rise. The correct breath volume is one that causes the chest to rise, without causing excessive gastric distension

11 While still maintaining head tilt and chin lift, remove your mouth and watch for chest fall, as the air comes out (Fig. 6.6)

12 Take another breath (pausing to take a breath will maximise the oxygen content and minimise the carbon dioxide content in the delivered breaths, and repeat steps 8–11

13 Deliver five initial breaths in total

Ineffective delivery of breaths

If it is difficult to deliver effective breaths:
- ensure adequate head tilt and chin lift
- reposition the airway (slight readjustment may be all that is required)
- recheck the child's mouth and remove any obstruction (no blind finger sweeps)
- ensure an airtight seal
- ensure the child's nose is pinched during ventilation
- try jaw thrust to open airway
- allow five attempts to achieve effective breaths. If still unsuccessful, proceed to chest compressions

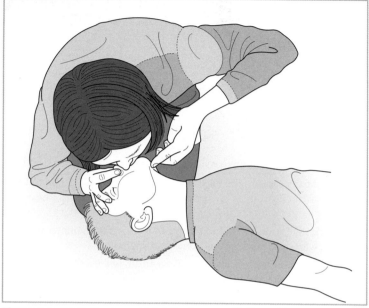

Figure 6.6 Ventilation in a child: following a ventilation, while still retaining head tilt and chin lift, remove the mouth and watch for chest fall, as the air comes out

Complications of gastric inflation

Gastric inflation is commonly associated with mouth-to-mouth ventilation, particularly if the rescue breaths are performed rapidly. It occurs when the pressure in the oesophagus exceeds the opening pressure of the lower oesophageal sphincter pressure, resulting in the sphincter opening. During CPR the oesophageal sphincter relaxes, thus increasing the likelihood of gastric inflation.

Complications of gastric inflation include:
* regurgitation
* aspiration
* pneumonia

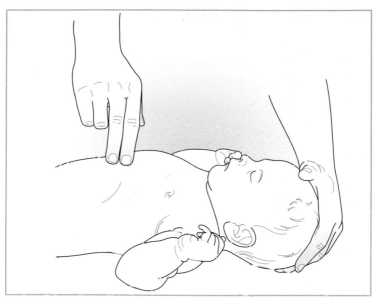

Figure 6.7 Chest compressions in an infant: two fingers on the lower third of the sternum

- diaphragm elevation, restricted lung movements and reduced lung compliance.

Gastric inflation can be minimised if rescue breaths are delivered slowly (over 1–1.5 seconds).

Principles of chest compressions

Chest compressions in an infant

Location: lower third of the sternum – two finger technique (Fig. 6.7); a more effective technique is the thumb technique, with the hands encircling the chest – this is the preferred method when two healthcare professionals are present (compression of the xiphoid process should be avoided as this may injure the liver, stomach or spleen).

Depth: one third of the depth of the chest (vertical pressure down) (see Fig. 3.9).

Rate: 100 per minute, coordinated with ventilations.

Ratio: 15 compressions: 2 ventilations (one rescuer would usually use 30:2 ratio)

Chest compressions in a child

Location: heel of one hand on the lower third of sternum

Depth: one third to one half of the depth of the chest (vertical pressure down) (Fig. 6.8).

Rate: 100 per minute.

Ratio: 15 compressions: 2 ventilations (one rescuer would usually use 30:2 ratio)

Chest compressions in an older child

In larger children it may be necessary to adopt the 'adult' two-handed technique for chest compressions (see Fig. 3.8), in order to achieve effective chest compressions.

Duration

Cerebral and coronary perfusion is optimum when 50% of the cycle is devoted to the chest compression phase and 50% to the chest relaxation phase.

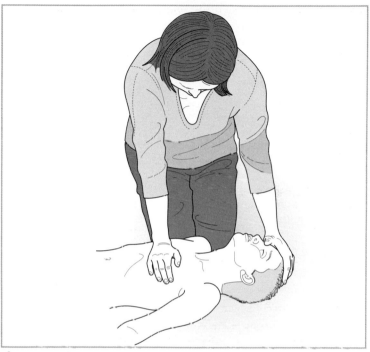

Figure 6.8 Chest compressions in a child: heel of one hand on the sternum, two fingers' breadth above the ziphisternum

Rate

A chest compression rate of 100 per minute is required to achieve optimum blood flow during CPR. The rate refers to the speed of compressions rather than the actual number delivered per minute. When chest compressions are interrupted to provide ventilations, the actual number delivered will therefore be <100 per minute and will vary from rescuer to rescuer, depending upon the time taken to position the head, open the airway and deliver the rescue breaths.

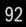
If the child is intubated by the paramedics, chest compressions and ventilations are asynchronous; the number of compressions delivered will then be approximately 100 per minute.

Recovery position

An unconscious child whose airway is clear, and who is breathing spontaneously, should be turned onto the side into the recovery position; this prevents the tongue falling back and obstructing the airway, and reduces the risk of inhalation of gastric contents.

Although there are a number of recovery positions currently advocated, no single one can be endorsed. However, the position adopted should:

- be stable
- maintain a patent airway
- maintain a stable cervical spine
- avoid application of pressure on the chest that restricts breathing
- minimise the risk of aspiration
- limit pressure on bony prominences and peripheral nerves
- enable visualisation of the child's breathing and colour
- allow access to the child for interventions
- be easy and safe to achieve (including repositioning if required).

Management of foreign body airway obstruction (FBAO)

Complete obstruction of the airway by a foreign body is a life-threatening emergency and is often characterised by a sudden inability to talk, maximal respiratory effort, development of cyanosis and clutching of the neck.

In partial airway obstruction, the child will be distressed, may cough and may have a wheeze. In complete airway obstruction, the child will be unable to speak, breathe or cough and will eventually become unconscious. The Resuscitation Council (UK) algorithm for the treatment of FBAO is detailed in Figure 6.9.

Treatment of FBAO in a conscious infant

The treatment algorithm for a choking infant, based on Resuscitation Council (UK) guidelines (2005) is depicted in Fig. 6.9.

If the infant is choking, but has an effective cough, encourage coughing and closely monitor. If the infant's cough is ineffective or becoming ineffective, shout out for help and:

1 Position the infant in a prone position resting on your forearm, with the head lower than the chest and the airway open. Ensure the head is well supported

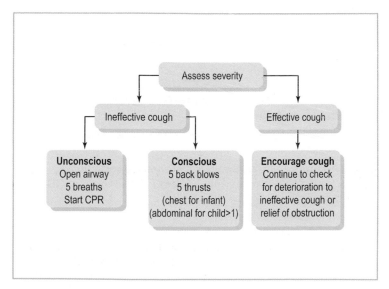

Fig. 6.9 Resuscitation Council (UK) paediatric foreign body airway obstruction treatment algorithm. Reproduced with permission from the Resuscitation Council (UK)

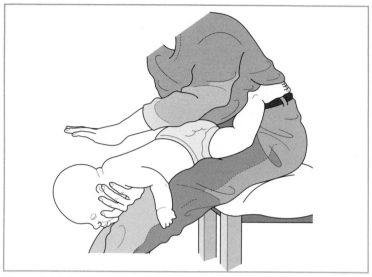

Figure 6.10 Relief of FBAO inan infants: back blows between the scapulae

2 Deliver up to five back blows between the scapulae using the heel of the hand (Fig. 6.10). If the back blows fail to dislodge the foreign body, proceed to chest thrusts

3 Turn the infant into a supine position, with the head lower than the chest and the airway open

4 Deliver up to five chest thrusts to the sternum (similar to chest compressions, but more vigorous, sharper and slower) (Fig. 6.11)

5 If the airway remains obstructed, repeat the sequence for back blows and chest thrusts as approriate.

6 If the infant becomes unconscious, open the airway, remove any obvious foreign body (no blind finger sweeps) and deliver five breaths. If there is no response proceed to chest compressions and perform CPR for 1 minute before alerting the emergency services (obviously if not alone, send another person to do this as soon as possible).

Abdominal thrusts are not recommended in infants

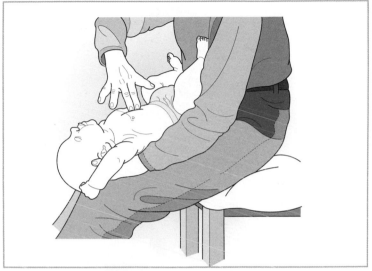

Figure 6.11 Infant choking on a foreign body: chest thrusts to the sternum

Treatment of FBAO in a conscious child

If the child is choking, but has an effective cough, encourage coughing and closely monitor. If the child's cough is ineffective or becoming ineffective, shout out for help and:

1 Position the child, with the head lower than the chest and the airway open. A small child could be placed across the lap.

2 Deliver up to five back blows between the scapulae using the heel of the hand. If the back blows fail to dislodge the foreign body, proceed to abdominal thrusts (Fig. 6.12)

3 Stand or kneel behind the child

4 Position your arms directly underneath the child's axillae and encircle the torso

5 Bend the child forward

6 Place the thumb side of one fist against the child's abdomen, between the umbilicus and the xiphoid process

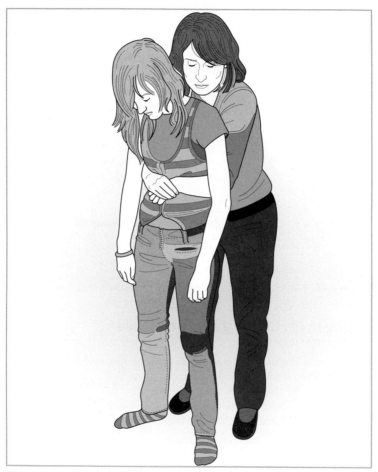

Figure 6.12 Relief of FBAO in a child (>1 year): abdominal thrusts

7 Grasp the fist with the other hand

8 Exert up to five quick inward and upward thrusts. Avoid touching the xiphoid process and lower margins of the rib cage because any force applied to these structures could damage internal organs

9 If the airway remains obstructed, repeat the sequence for back blows and abdominal thrusts as appropriate

10 If the child becomes unconscious, open the airway, remove any obvious foreign body (no blind finger sweeps) and deliver five breaths. If there is no response, proceed to chest compressions and perform CPR for 1 minute before alerting the emergency services (obviously if not alone, send another person to do this as soon as possible)

If teaching a lay person the management of foreign body airway obstruction, it is recommended to advise that CPR should be undertaken for 1 minute and then the emergency services activated if a choking infant or child loses consciousness. This is because chest compressions could generate sufficient pressure to remove a foreign body.

Conclusion

Cardiopulmonary arrests in infants and children are usually secondary to either respiratory or circulatory failure, and rarely result from a primary cardiac event. Respiratory failure is the most common cause and effective oxygenation and ventilation must be established as quickly as possible. This chapter has provided an overview of the principles of paediatric BLS.

Anaphylaxis

Anaphylaxis

Introduction

Anaphylaxis is a severe systemic allergic reaction involving respiratory difficulty and/or hypotension, with other clinical features possibly present as well. It can be life-threatening because of the rapid onset of airway compromise due to laryngeal oedema, respiratory difficulties due to severe bronchoconstriction and/or the development of cardiovascular collapse and profound shock. Between 1992 and 2001 there were 214 deaths attributed to anaphylaxis in the UK (Pumphrey, 2004).

The incidence of anaphylaxis is increasing, probably linked to an appreciable rise in the prevalence of allergic disease over the last 20–30 years. Between 1990/91 and 2000/01 there were 13 250 hospital admissions for anaphylaxis in England.

'The management of anaphylaxis includes early recognition, anticipation of deterioration, and aggressive support of airway, oxygenation, ventilation, and circulation' (AHA & ILCOR, 2000). In the community setting the priority is, therefore, to call an ambulance.

The aim of this chapter is to understand the first aid treatment of anaphylaxis.

Chapter objectives
At the end of the chapter the reader will be able to:

- List the common causes of anaphylaxis

- Discuss the signs and symptoms of anaphylaxis

- Describe the treatment of anaphylaxis in adults

- Describe the treatment of anaphylaxis in children

- Describe the use of adrenaline (epinephrine) auto-injector device

Common causes of anaphylaxis

Common causes of anaphylaxis include:

- peanuts and tree nuts: commonest cause of food-related anaphylaxis; in the UK 1:200 people have peanut allergy. The main danger with peanut-induced anaphylaxis is the development of laryngeal oedema. Peanuts and nuts account for 94% of fatal and near-fatal anaphylactic reactions to food

- fish, shell-fish and shrimps

- insect venom: e.g. bee or wasp stings

- penicillin: accounts for most drug-induced anaphylaxis episodes

- aspirin and non-steroidal anti-inflammatory drugs (NSAID) and fatalities are possible

- latex: important cause of occupational allergy; latex allergy is usually of a slower onset (30 minutes) because the allergen is absorbed through the skin; latex is present in a number of household products including balloons, rubber bands, carpet backing, Lycra in clothes, furniture filling and elastic in clothing

- exercise: often requires both exercise and ingestion of particular foods

- vaccinations.

Signs and symptoms of anaphylaxis

Anaphylaxis can vary in severity (mild to life-threatening). The onset following allergen exposure can be sudden, but sometimes delayed, and the progress can be slow, rapid or even biphasic. Signs and symptoms include:

- bronchospasm: cough, chest tightness, dyspnoea and wheeze

- laryngeal oedema: hoarseness, dysphagia, 'lump in throat', drooling, stridor, asphyxia; oedema of the lips, tongue, soft palate and uvula may herald concomitant laryngeal oedema

- circulatory shock: light-headedness, dizziness, syncope, agitation, tachycardia, pallor, hypotension

- urticaria: pruritus, flushing, raised wheals on the skin

- angioedema: tingling and swollen sensation
- conjunctivitis
- gastroenteritis: symptoms include colic, abdominal cramps, diarrhoea and vomiting.

Treatment of anaphylaxis in adults

The treatment of anaphylaxis is difficult to standardise because aetiology, clinical presentation (including severity and course) and organ involvement can vary widely. The Consensus guidelines for the emergency treatment of anaphylaxis in adults in the community are outlined in the algorithm in Figure 7.1, which provides a structural and systematic approach based on current recommendations (The Project Team of the Resuscitation Council (UK), 2005). The algorithm takes into account the probable limited facilities, equipment and drugs in the community setting and stresses the:

- urgency of arranging hospital transfer
- need for administering adrenaline (epinephrine) promptly if there is stridor, wheeze, respiratory stress or clinical features of shock.

Diagnosis

Early intervention is critical to the successful management of anaphylaxis. It is therefore paramount promptly to recognise the signs and symptoms of anaphylaxis and treat it quickly and effectively. Consider the diagnosis of anaphylaxis when there is a history suggestive of an allergic-type reaction with respiratory difficulty and/or hypotension, particularly if there are skin changes present.

Getting help

As soon as anaphylaxis is suspected, alert the emergency services and suggest a diagnosis.

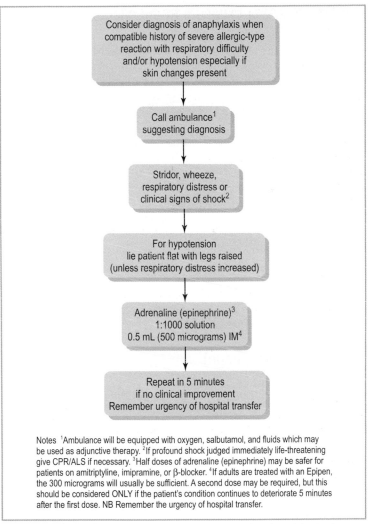

Consider diagnosis of anaphylaxis when
compatible history of severe allergic-type
reaction with respiratory difficulty
and/or hypotension especially if
skin changes present

Call ambulance[1]
suggesting diagnosis

Stridor, wheeze,
respiratory distress or
clinical signs of shock[2]

For hypotension
lie patient flat with legs raised
(unless respiratory distress increased)

Adrenaline (epinephrine)[3]
1:1000 solution
0.5 mL (500 micrograms) IM[4]

Repeat in 5 minutes
if no clinical improvement
Remember urgency of hospital transfer

Notes [1]Ambulance will be equipped with oxygen, salbutamol, and fluids which may
be used as adjunctive therapy. [2]If profound shock judged immediately life-threatening
give CPR/ALS if necessary. [3]Half doses of adrenaline (epinephrine) may be safer for
patients on amitriptyline, imipramine, or β-blocker. [4]If adults are treated with an Epipen,
the 300 micrograms will usually be sufficient. A second dose may be required, but this
should be considered ONLY if the patient's condition continues to deteriorate 5 minutes
after the first dose. NB Remember the urgency of hospital transfer.

Figure 7.1 Anaphylactic reactions: treatment algorithm for adults in the
community. Reproduced with permission from Aurum Pharmaceuticals

Preventing further exposure to the allergen

If possible, prevent further administration and absorption of the allergen, e.g. bee sting, scrape any insect parts off the skin, but do not squeeze them as this allegedly increases envenomation.

Casualty position

Recline the casualty into a comfortable position. If the casualty is hypotensive, lay the casualty flat and elevate the legs (unless respiratory distress is increased).

There have been reported cases of casualties in anaphylactic shock who, following a change to a more upright position, have developed cardiac arrest.

Oxygen

If available, administer high flow rates of oxygen as it is an important adjunctive therapy.

Adrenaline (epinephrine)

Adrenaline (epinephrine) is the most important drug in severe anaphylaxis.

The beneficial effects of adrenaline (epinephrine) include:
- peripheral vasoconstriction which will help to increase the blood pressure and reduce angioedema of the skin and mucous membranes
- bronchodilation
- increase in myocardial contractility
- prevention of the further release of chemical mediators, e.g. histamine from mast cells.

If available, administer adrenaline (epinephrine) 500 µg IM if there is stridor, wheeze, respiratory distress or there are clinical features of shock (Project Team of the Resuscitation Council (UK), 2005), following local policy. It is almost always effective, when administered promptly.

Indications for adrenaline (epinephrine): stridor, wheeze, respiratory distress or clinical features of shock (The Project Team of the Resuscitation Council (UK), 2005)

The recommended dose is 500 µg (0.5 ml of 1:1000 solution) IM into the thigh, which can be repeated after 5 minutes if there is no improvement or if deterioration has occurred, particularly if the casualty's conscious level becomes, or remains, impaired in the presence of hypotension (Resuscitation Council (UK), 2001). A lower dose may be safer in some situations (e.g. patient prescribed tricyclics).

Use of adrenaline (epinephrine) auto-injector device

An adrenaline (epinephrine) auto-injector device is designed for immediate self-administration by a person with a history of anaphylaxis. It is intended as emergency supportive treatment only, and is not a substitute for seeking medical help (immediately); urgent transfer to hospital is paramount. If the casualty has a device assist with its use.

There are currently two auto-injector devices licensed in the UK for self-administration of adrenaline (epinephrine): EpiPen (Alk Abello) (Fig. 7.2) and Anapen (Celltech) (Fig. 7.3). Both devices are fully assembled syringes that can deliver a single dose of adrenaline (epinephrine) 300 µg IM. Paediatric versions are also available: EpiPen Jr and Anapen Junior, each able to deliver a single dose of 150 µg.

The Project Team of the Resuscitation Council UK (2005) suggest:
- The 150 µg device can be administered in children from 6 months to 6 years (instead of 120 µg)

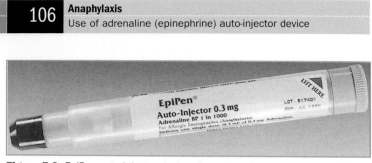

Figure 7.2 EpiPen auto-injector device. Reproduced with permission from Alk-Abelló Ltd

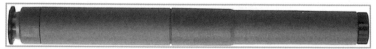

Figure 7.3 Anapen auto-injector device. Reproduced with permission from Lincoln Medical Ltd

- The 300 µg device can be administered in children >6 years (instead of 250 µg or 500 µg).

Operating the EpiPen

The procedure for operating the EpiPen is as follows:
1 Remove the EpiPen from the packaging
2 Grasp the Epipen in the dominant hand, with thumb closest to the grey safety cap
3 With the other hand, pull off the grey safety cap (Fig. 7.4A)
4 Hold EpiPen approximately 10 cm away from the outer thigh; the black tip should point towards the outer thigh (Fig. 7.4B)
5 Jab firmly into the outer thigh so that the EpiPen is at right angles to the outer thigh, through the clothing if necessary (Fig. 7.4C)
6 Hold the EpiPen in place for 10 seconds
7 Remove the EpiPen and massage the area for 10 seconds (Alk Abello, 2005).

Although 'fluid' can still be seen in the auto-injector after use, the unit cannot be used again. The EpiPen should be disposed of following the manufacturer's recommendations.

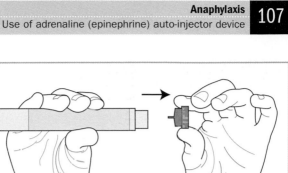
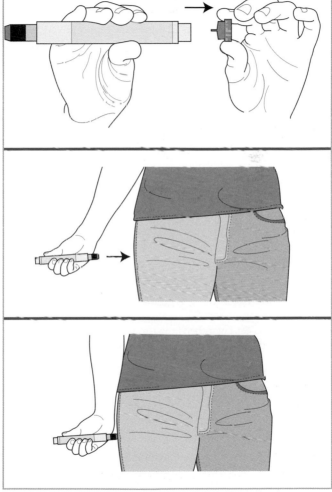

Figure 7.4 Using the EpiPen: place the black tip at right angles to the thigh and press hard until the auto-injector mechanism functions (there should be a click). Reproduced with permission from Alk Abello Ltd (UK)

Operating the Anapen

The procedure for operating the Anapen is as follows:

1 Remove the black needle cap. This pulls the rubber protective sheath off the needle

2 Remove the black safety cap from the red firing button

3 Hold the needle end of the device against the outer thigh. If necessary, the injection may be made through light clothing

4 Press the firing button. A spring-activated plunger pushes the needle into the muscle and injects the full dose of adrenaline (epinephrine) (Fig. 7.5)

5 Hold the device in position for 10 seconds, then remove it

6 Gently massage the injection site for approximately 10 seconds

7 Replace the black needle cap and discard the device safely immediately after use (Celltech Pharmaceuticals product literature).

Other treatments

Other treatments which the emergency services will probably administer include:

• an antihistamine, e.g. chlorphenamine, to help counteract the histamine-mediated vasodilation and relieve the cutaneous manifestations of urticaria

• a corticosteroid to help prevent late sequelae

• IV fluids, if severe hypotension fails to respond rapidly to drug therapy.

• beta 2 agonist nebuliser

Inhaled beta 2 agonist

A beta 2 agonist is indicated if bronchoconstriction is a prominent feature that is not responding to conventional treatment (Project Team of the Resuscitation Council (UK), 2002). If the casualty has a beta 2 inhaler and has a wheeze it would be sensible to suggest its use.

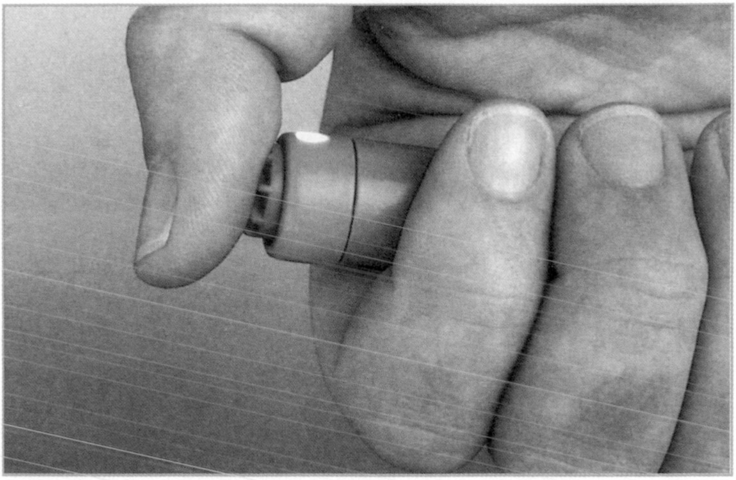

Figure 7.5 Using the Anapen: hold the needle end of the device against the outer thigh, press the firing button: a spring-activated plunger pushes the needle into the muscle and injects the full dose of adrenaline (epinephrine). Reproduced with permission from Lincoln Medical Ltd

Life-threatening airway obstruction

Of particular concern is the potential rapid progression to life-threatening airway obstruction and asphyxia. While waiting for the emergency services continually monitor the casualty's vital signs. Angioedema of the uvula, tongue, soft palate or lips could indicate concomitant laryngeal oedema. The presence of hoarseness, dysphagia, lump in the throat, stridor and drooling suggests the development of laryngeal oedema.

Assessment and re-assessment

While awaiting the emergency services, monitor the casualty's vital signs:

- airway: patency
- breathing: mechanics, efficacy and adequacy

- circulation: pulse rate, skin colour
- conscious level: AVPU.

The patency of the upper airway and the casualty's haemodynamic status should be closely monitored because laryngeal oedema (causing asphyxia) and shock are principal causes of death associated with anaphylaxis.

Psychological care

An anaphylaxis episode will be very frightening and anxiety may exacerbate the effects of anaphylaxis; reassure the casualty.

Post-anaphylaxis management

Both during and after an anaphylactic reaction it is most important to monitor the casualty closely. This involves assessment and constant re-assessment of the casualty's vital signs. The patency of the upper airway and the casualty's haemodynamic status should also be closely monitored.

Sometimes the initial reaction is then followed by a late-phase reaction, which usually begins after 2–4 hours, peaks between 6 and 12 hours and resolves within 24–48 hours. This late-phase or biphasic reaction can be even more profound than the first.

Measurement of mast cell tryptase

Measurement of mast cell tryptase can help with the retrospective diagnosis of anaphylaxis. Serum tryptase levels are raised in the immediate period (maximum level at 60 minutes) following an anaphylactic reaction. Serum levels of tryptase correlate linearly with the severity of the symptoms.

Indications for admission

Biphasic reactions are not uncommon, particularly in patients who require higher doses of adrenaline (epinephrine) initially to control their symptoms. Sometimes close monitoring for 8–24 hours will be required, particularly when the reaction:

- is severe and is of slow onset due to idiopathic anaphylaxis
- occurs in a severe asthmatic
- is complicated by a severe asthmatic attack
- could be triggered again because further absorption of the allergen is possible
(Project Team of the Resuscitation Council (UK), 2005).

Even if the casualty responds to treatment, there is a risk of a second phase reaction. Consideration will need to be given to later assessment and management. Therefore encourage the casualty to seek medical help.

Later assessment and management

The casualty should be referred to an allergist, preferably one with experience in anaphylaxis. The aim of later assessment is to identify/confirm the causative allergen where possible and to educate the casualty and general practitioner regarding future allergen avoidance and the appropriate management of any future episodes of anaphylaxis. The casualty may also require an adrenaline (epinephrine) auto-injector device.

Conclusion

Anaphylaxis is a severe systemic allergic reaction. It can be life-threatening because of the rapid onset of airway compromise due to laryngeal oedema, respiratory difficulties due to severe bronchoconstriction and/or the development of cardiovascular collapse and profound shock. In the community setting the priority is therefore to call an ambulance. The use of an adrenaline (epinephrine) auto-injector device can be life-saving.

Respiratory problems

Respiratory problems

Introduction

Problems affecting the respiratory system can be life-threatening. It is important to assess the casualty's vital signs, particularly respiratory function (see pp. 20–22) and then take appropriate action. If possible, identify and remove the cause of the problem and provide fresh air. Continually monitor the casualty as basic life support (BLS) may be required.

The aim of this chapter is to understand the first aid treatment of respiratory problems.

Chapter objectives
At the end of the chapter the reader will be able to discuss the treatment for:

- **Acute asthma**

- **Hyperventilation**

- **Smoke and toxic fumes inhalation**

- **Open chest wound**

- **Hanging and strangulation**

- **Near-drowning**

- **Diving accidents**

Acute asthma

Asthma can be defined as:

a chronic inflammatory disorder of the airways ... in susceptible individuals, inflammatory symptoms are usually associated with widespread but variable airway obstruction and an increase in airway response to a variety of stimuli. Obstruction is often reversible, either spontaneously or with treatment (British Thoracic Society & Scottish Intercollegiate Guidelines Network (BTS & SIGN), 2004).

The incidence of acute asthma episodes in primary care is on the decline.

The speed of the onset of an acute attack can vary; although it can come on over a period of minutes, there has usually been a background of deterioration over a period of days or weeks. A helpful guide indicating deterioration is the need to use bronchodilator inhalers more frequently than normal or that they are less effective. The severity of acute asthma can range from moderate to life-threatening (Fig. 8.1).

Factors increasing the risk of life-threatening asthma

Factors increasing the risk of life-threatening asthma include:
- previous ventilation
- admission to hospital with asthma in the previous 12 months
- frequent rescue medication use
- three classes of asthma medication
- repeated attendances in A & E with asthma
- brittle asthma
  (Ramrakha & Moore, 2004).

MANAGEMENT OF ACUTE ASTHMA IN ADULTS

ASSESSMENT OF SEVERE ASTHMA

B Healthcare professionals must be aware that patients with severe asthma and one or more adverse psychosocial factors (psychiatric illness, alcohol or drug abuse, denial, unemployment, etc) are at risk of death

☑ • Keep patients who have had near fatal asthma or brittle asthma under specialist supervision indefinitely
• A respiratory specialist should follow up patients admitted with severe asthma for at least one year after admission

INITIAL ASSESSMENT

MODERATE EXACERBATION

• increasing symptoms
• PEF >50–75% best or predicted
• no features of acute severe asthma

ACUTE SEVERE

Any one of:
• PEF 33–50% best or predicted
• respiratory rate ≥25/min
• heart rate ≥110/min
• inability to complete sentences in one breath

LIFE THREATENING

In a patient with severe asthma any one of:
• PEF <33% best or predicted
• SpO_2 <92%
• PaO_2 <8 kPa
• normal $PaCO_2$ (4.6–6.0 kPa)
• silent chest
• cyanosis
• feeble respiratory effort
• bradycardia, dysrhythmia, hypotension
• exhaustion, confusion, coma

NEAR FATAL

Raised $PaCO_2$ and/or requiring mechanical ventilation with raised inflation pressures

■ Applies only to adults ■ Applies to children 5–12 ■ Applies to children under 5 ■ General

Figure 8.1 Severity of acute asthma. Reproduced with permission from British Guideline on the Management of Asthma

MANAGEMENT OF ACUTE ASTHMA IN ADULTS	
Clinical features	Severe breathlessness (including too breathless to complete sentences in one breath), tachypriea, tachycardina, silent chest, cyanosis or collapse *None of these singly or together is specific and their absence does not exclude a severe attack*
PEF or FEV1	PFF or FEV1 are useful and valid measures of airway calibre. PEF expressed as a % of patient's previous best value is most useful clinically. In the absence of this, PEF as a % of predicted is a rough guide
Pulse oximetry	Oxygen saturation (SpO2) measured by pulse oximetry determines the adequacy of oxygen therapy and the need for arterial blood gas (ABG). The aim of oxygen therapy is to maintain SpO2 ≥92%
Blood gases (ABG)	Patients with SpO2 <92% or other features of life-threatening asthma require ABG measurement
Chest X-ray	Chest X-ray is not routinely recommended in the absence of: • suspected pneumomediastinum or pneumothorax • suspected consolidation • life-threatening asthma • failure to respond to treatment satisfactorily • requirement for ventilation

Applies only to adults ■ Applies to children 5–12 Applies to children under 5 General

Figure 8.1 *(cont'd)*

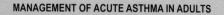

MANAGEMENT OF ACUTE ASTHMA IN ADULTS

CRITERIA FOR ADMISSION

B Admit patients with any feature of
- a life-threatening or near-fatal attack
- severe attack persisting after initial treatment

C Patients whose peak flow is greater than 75% best or predicted one hour after initial treatment may be discharged from A&E, unless there are other reasons why admission may be appropriate

TREATMENT OF ACUTE ASTHMA

OXYGEN

C • Give high flow oxygen to all patients with acute asthma

A • Nebulised β_2 agonist bronchodilators should be driven by oxygen (hospital, ambulance and primary care

C • The non-availability of supplemental oxygen should not prevent nebulised therapy being given if indicated

β_2 AGONIST BRONCHODILATORS

A Administer high dose inhaled β_2 agonists as first line agents and administer as early as possible. Outside hospital high dose β_2 agonist bronchodilators may be delivered via large volume spacer or nebuliser

☑ In acute asthma with life-threatening features the nebulised route (oxygen-driven) is recommended

A In severe asthma (PEF or FEV_1 <50% best or predicted) and asthma that is poorly responsive to an initial bolus dose of β_2 agonist, consider continuous nebulisation

Applies only to adults ■ Applies to children 5–12 Applies to children under 5 General

Figure 8.1 *(cont'd)*

MANAGEMENT OF ACUTE ASTHMA IN ADULTS

STEROID THERAPY

A Give systemic steroids in adequate doses in all cases

☑ Continue prednisolone 40–50 mg daily for at least 5 days or until recovery

OTHER THERAPIES

A Consider a single dose of IV magnesium sulphate (1.2–2 g IV infusion over 20 minutes) for patients with:
- acute severe asthma without a good initial response to inhaled broncho-dilator therapy
- life-threatening or near-fatal asthma

☑ IV magnesium sulphate should only be used following consultation with senior medical staff

B Routine prescription of antibiotics is not recommended

IPRATROPIUM BROMIDE

A Nebulised ipratropium bromide (0.5 mg 4–6 hourly) should be added to β2 agonist treatment for patients with acute severe or life-threatening asthma or those with a poor initial response to β2 agonist therapy

REFERRAL TO INTENSIVE CARE

Refer any patient:
- requiring ventilatory support
- with acute severe or life-threatening asthma, failing to respond to therapy, evidenced by:
  - deteriorating PEF
  - persisting or worsening hypoxia
  - hypercapnia
  - ABG analysis showing ↓pH or ↑H+
  - exhaustion, feeble respiration
  - drowsiness, confusion
  - coma or respiratory arrest

Applies only to adults ■ Applies to children 5–12   Applies to children under 5   General

Figure 8.1 *(cont'd)*

Factors contributing to a poor outcome

Factors contributing to a poor outcome include:
- doctors failing to assess severity by objective measurement
- patients or relatives failing to recognise the severity of an attack
- under-use of corticosteroids (British Thoracic Society & Scottish Intercollegiate Guidelines Network (BTS & SIGN), 2004).

Many asthma-related deaths are preventable, but delay can be fatal (BTS & SIGN, 2004). Mortality is most often associated with failure to appreciate the severity of the exacerbation, resulting in inadequate emergency treatment and delay in referring to hospital (Rodrigo et al, 2004).

Signs and symptoms

Signs and symptoms of asthma include:
- wheeze
- shortness of breath
- chest tightness
- cough.

The hallmark of asthma is that these symptoms tend to be:
- variable
- intermittent
- worse at night
- provoked by triggers including exercise.

Patients with severe or life-threatening asthma may not be distressed

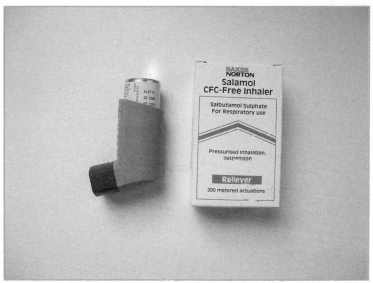

Figure 8.2 Relief inhaler

Treatment

- Assess the casualty's respiratory function
- Sit the casualty up
- If available, consult the casualty's individual action plan in the event of an asthma attack
- Encourage the casualty to take his relief inhaler (Fig. 8.2)
- Ask the casualty to breathe slowly and deeply
- Monitor the casualty's vital signs, particularly respiratory rate, heart rate and conscious level
- Record peak expiratory flow (PEF) if the casualty has PEF meter (Fig. 8.3); document the result
- Reassure the casualty; an acute attack of asthma is frightening and hospital transfer may increase anxiety and exacerbate symptoms; reassurance that treatment is available to relieve the attack is an important aspect of care

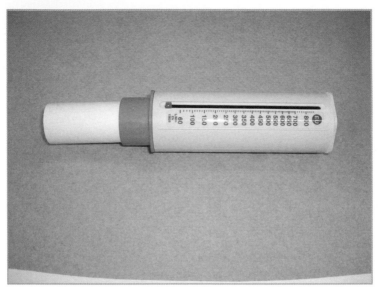

Figure 8.3 Peak expiratory flow (PEF) meter. Reproduced with permission from Clement Clark International

Indications for hospital admission

Asthma has been classified into moderate, severe and life-threatening (see Fig. 8.1). For moderate, severe and asthma, the following is recommended:

Moderate asthma: treat at home or in the surgery and assess response to treatment.

Severe asthma: immediate transfer to hospital should be arranged if the casualty is not responding to treatment.

Life-threatening asthma: immediate transfer to hospital should be arranged.

Factors lowering the threshold for hospital admission include:
- afternoon or evening attack
- recent nocturnal symptoms
- recent hospital admission
- previous severe attacks
- casualty unable to assess own condition
- concern regarding social circumstances
  (Rees & Kanabar, 2000; BTS & SIGN, 2005).

Hyperventilation

Hyperventilation is usually anxiety induced and may accompany a panic attack. It can occur in a susceptible individual who has recently experienced emotional or psychological trauma. It can lead to hypocapnia, causing tingling in the extremities and the mouth, dizziness, trembling and cramps.

Treatment

- Reassure the casualty
- If possible remove the cause of the distress/anxiety
- Ensure privacy
- Encourage the casualty to breathe normally and regain control of breathing

If still hyperventilating, ask the casualty to breathe into a paper bag:
- Ensure the paper bag covers the casualty's nose and mouth (Fig. 8.4)
- Ask the casualty to breathe in and out slowly about 10 times
- Then ask the casualty to breathe without the paper bag for 15 seconds
- Alternate this cycle of breathing until the hyperventilation has stopped (St John Ambulance, 2002).

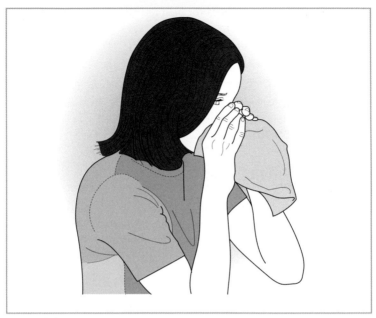

Figure 8.4 Hyperventilation: using a paper bag

Smoke and toxic fumes inhalation

Smoke inhalation can cause a combination of thermal and chemical injury to the respiratory system, with varying degrees of systemic toxicity. In casualties with smoke inhalation, the main cause of mortality is cerebral hypoxia secondary to exposure to carbon monoxide.

Toxic fumes can be generated by the combustion of household materials:
- sulphur dioxide and nitrogen dioxide (wood and petroleum)
- hydrochloric acid (polyvinyl chloride)

- toluene diisocyanate (polyurethane)
  (Ramrakha & Moore, 2004).

Clinical features

Clinical features include:
- cough
- sore throat
- dyspnoea
- pleuritic retrosternal chest pain
- headache
- dizziness
- nausea
  (Ramrakha & Moore, 2004).

Treatment

- Alert the emergency services
- If the casualty is burning, attempt to extinguish the flames (see p. 11)
- Move the casualty away from the source of the smoke/fumes to a place of fresh air
- Loosen any tight clothing worn by the casualty
- Support and reassure the casualty and assist to breathe normally
- Monitor the casualty's vital signs, particularly breathing – note any signs of developing airway compromise due to inhalation injury
- High flow oxygen is indicated at the earliest opportunity

Thermal inhalation injury

Thermal inhalation injury is a major source of morbidity and mortality, particularly when associated with a burn injury within a confined space. Clinical features and treatment of thermal inhalation injury to the respiratory tract are discussed on page 22.

Open chest wound

An open chest wound or 'sucking wound' can be caused by a
penetrating chest wound, a bomb injury or blast injury. The prime
object, while maintaining cardiorespiratory function, is to seal this
wound.

Treatment

- Sit the casualty down
- Encourage the casualty to lean towards the injured side
- Place a sterile dressing over the wound and cover with plastic
- Seal the plastic with tape on three sides only, ensuring it is taut, leaving
  the lower side free. This will create a makeshift 'flutter valve', allowing
  air to be released under pressure, i.e. on expiration, but not drawn into
  the pleural cavity during inspiration

Hanging and strangulation

Both hanging and strangulation involve compression of the trachea
and major blood vessels in the neck.

Hanging: the body is suspended by a noose around the neck and
there may be a serious injury to the cervical spine. Particular care
and attention is required to minimise the risk of aggravating the
injury. Deliberate hanging is a form of attempted suicide.

Strangulation: constriction around the neck may be caused by
accident, e.g. an item of clothing, such as a tie, becoming caught in
machinery. Infants and young children are particularly vulnerable
to accidental strangulation by items such as cot rails, bib straps,
banisters and rails. An accidental atypical hanging with the collar
of a sweater has been reported (Nurhantari et al, 2002).

Survival from hanging or strangulation can be associated with
various complications, including a large variety of neurological

consequences. Poor prognostic indicators of hanging include prolonged hanging time, unconsciousness and cardiac arrest at the scene.

Signs and symptoms

* Constricting item around the neck
* Numerous tiny haemorrhages above the constriction line and on the whites of the eyes
* Congestion of the face, with very prominent veins
* Rapid and laboured breathing due to constriction and swelling around the neck

Treatment

It is imperative to remove the constricting item and provide first aid as quickly as possible to optimise the chances of successful resuscitation. The following is recommended:

* call out for help
* quickly remove any constriction from around the neck of the casualty; if still hanging, support the body while this is being done. (NB The body may be very heavy.) It may be necessary to cut the rope or constricting article from around the neck (Fig. 8.5). Leave the knot intact as this may be required by the police.
* lay the casualty on the floor and assess ABC; assessment of the casualty may be difficult due to gross oedema of the neck and face which can make airway assessment and carotid pulse palpation very difficult
* start BLS if required (take care with the neck)
* do not move the casualty unnecessarily, in case there is a spinal injury
* ensure the emergency services are called, even if the casualty appears to make a full recovery (St John Ambulance, 2002).

The incident may need to be investigated by the police. It is important to ensure that potential evidence, e.g. the rope or piece of clothing found around the casualty's neck, is not destroyed

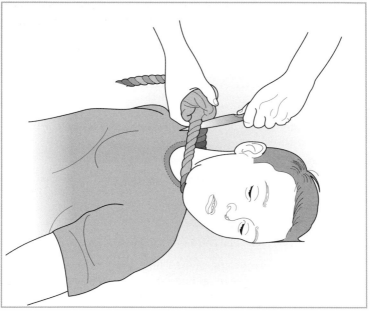

Figure 8.5 Hanging/strangulation: it may be necessary to cut the rope or constricting article from around the neck

Near-drowning

Drowning is defined as death by asphyxia due to submersion in a liquid medium, while near-drowning is defined as immediate survival after asphyxia due to submersion. Drowning is a frequent preventable accident that is associated with significant morbidity and mortality in a mostly healthy population.

Pathophysiology

Wet drowning: water enters the lungs and rapidly causes respiratory failure and cardiac arrest.

Dry drowning: a small amount of inhaled water causes the upper airways to go into spasm, leading to asphyxia and cardiac arrest.

Cold shock: once the casualty falls into cold water, he takes an automatic and involuntary gasp and starts hyperventilating.

Statistics

Water immersion is a frequent cause of accidental death and hospital admission. Some relevant facts:

- 450 people drown each year in the UK (more common in males)
- 60 children under 15 drown each year; drowning is among the leading causes of death in children under 5 years of age
- drowning is the third commonest cause of accidental death in children
- most drowning events happen in rivers, lakes and reservoirs
- often, casualties have forgotten to take safety precautions
- many drownings are linked to the use or abuse of alcohol
- activities frequently related to drowning included boating, falling, swimming and activities on ice.

The characteristics of drowning episodes vary greatly by age; in older children and adults most drowning episodes occur in open water. In most casualties, the primary injury is pulmonary, resulting in severe arterial hypoxaemia and secondary damage to other organs.

Central nervous system damage is most critical in terms of casualty survival and subsequent quality of life; prompt resuscitation is paramount. Case studies have convincingly demonstrated that near-drowning casualties can survive neurologically intact even after prolonged submersion times, particularly in cold water.

Treatment

> If the casualty had dived into shallow water there may be a cervical spine injury

- Try to rescue the casualty without entering the water; water rescue is a skilled operation for trained personnel (see pp. 11–13 Water rescue)
- Ensure the emergency services are alerted (even if the casualty appears to have recovered – secondary drowning can occur several hours later)
- Remove wet clothes if possible and keep the casualty warm
- If the casualty is breathing, place in the recovery position, ideally with the head low down so that water drains from the mouth

Manoeuvres to 'drain the lungs' are ineffective and potentially dangerous

Diving accidents

Air embolism

An air embolism can occur if the diver's breath is held on ascent; this can lead to an expansion of the volume of gas in the lungs, resulting in steep pressure gradients and alveoli rupture. Ruptured pulmonary veins can lead to arterial air embolism, usually into the carotid circulation.

Signs and symptoms

Clinical features could include:
- changes in behaviour
- confusion
- seizures
- coma
- cardiopulmonary arrest.

Treatment

- If there is a possibility of an air embolism, lie the casualty on the left side with head-down tilt to collect air in the right atrium
- Monitor the casualty's vital signs
- Ensure the emergency services are alerted
- Do not administer nitrous oxide (Entonox)

Decompression illness

Following a dive, a rapid ascent can lead to the formation of bubbles as dissolved nitrogen in the plasma comes out of solution.

Signs and symptoms

Signs and symptoms, which usually present within the first hour of surfacing, include:

- deep muscle aches ('the bends')
- painful, itching and burning skin
- retrosternal pain, cough and dyspnoea
- neurological symptoms, e.g. paraplegia, urinary retention (Ramrakha & Moore, 2004).

Treatment

- Alert the emergency services
- Immediate recompression will be required
- Minimise movement and high flow oxygen will be required.

Conclusion

In this chapter problems affecting the respiratory system have been discussed. It is important to assess the casualty's vital signs and take appropriate action. Be prepared to provided BLS if needed. If possible identify and remove the cause of the problem and provide fresh air.

Cardiac and circulatory problems

Cardiac and circulatory problems

Introduction

Ischaemic heart disease (IHD) is a leading cause of death in the western world. A characteristic symptom of IHD is chest pain. Chest pain is the commonest reason for alerting the emergency services; 10% of casualties taken to hospital with chest pain have had an acute myocardial infarction (MI). If a casualty has chest pain, it is essential to ensure that the appropriate management is given.

The term 'acute coronary syndrome (ACS)' is now commonly used to describe acute MI and unstable angina, because they both have in common a ruptured atheromatous plaque (American Heart Association, 2000). In the first aid situation, it is important to ascertain whether the casualty may have unstable angina or may be having an acute MI, as both require urgent transfer to hospital and investigations to help confirm the diagnosis, establish the immediate risk and determine the most appropriate treatment.

The aim of this chapter is to understand the first aid treatment for cardiac and circulatory problems.

Chapter objectives
At the end of the chapter the reader will be able to discuss the first aid treatment of:

- Angina

- Myocardial infarction

- Palpitations

- Shock

Angina

Angina occurs when there is an increase in myocardial oxygen demand that cannot be met by coronary supply. There is often a history of angina and risk factors include smoking, hypercholesterolaemia, hypertension, diabetes mellitus or a family history of ischaemic heart disease under the age of 60 years.

Precipitants

Precipitants of angina include:
* exercise, particularly climbing stairs or an incline
* emotion, particularly anger or anxiety
* a large meal – can increase cardiac output by 20%
* cold, windy weather
* exciting programmes on television – 'Match of the Day' angina
* life-like, frightening dreams
* sexual intercourse, particularly if extramarital or with a new partner (British Heart Foundation, 2005).

Signs and symptoms

Typical signs and symptoms include:
* retrosternal chest pain; crushing in nature, often described as a tight 'band' or 'vice'
* pain can radiate into the neck, throat, jaw, back and down one or both arms (usually inner side of arm, under the axilla to the inner two fingers) (British Heart Foundation, 2005).

Treatment

* Encourage the casualty to sit down and rest
* If the casualty has a GTN spray help in its use
* Reassure the casualty

- Monitor the severity of the pain: if it is not relieved by rest and medication after 15 minutes alert the emergency services (British Heart Foundation, 2005)

When to alert the emergency services

Alert the emergency services if:
- the chest pain lasts longer than 15 minutes and is not eased with rest or GTN spray as he may be having an acute coronary syndrome (ACS), i.e. unstable angina or acute MI
- the chest pain recurs, as he may be having an ACS (British Heart Foundation, 2005).

Myocardial infarction

In the UK alone, over 270 000 people each year have an MI (Resuscitation Council UK and British Heart Foundation, 2003). MI, or 'heart attack' as it is sometimes termed, is the leading cause of death in the UK.

Fifty per cent of sudden cardiac deaths occur within the first hour of onset, and 75% within 3 hours of onset of an acute MI. The most common cause of death is ventricular fibrillation. The risk of this, together with the life-saving benefits of coronary reperfusion therapy (see below), reinforces the urgency of ensuring that the emergency services are alerted and the casualty transferred speedily to hospital for urgent assessment.

There are two practical methods of coronary reperfusion therapy: thrombolytic therapy and percutaneous transluminal coronary angioplasty (PTCA). The benefits of thrombolytic therapy in the management of an acute MI are well known: a recent overview of all randomised trials showed a short-term reduction in mortality of 24% (AHA & ILCOR, 2000). The effect on mortality has been shown to continue for up to 10 years (GISSI, 1998). In some areas of the UK, thrombolytic therapy will be started by the emergency services. Some patients are admitted directly for PTCA.

Aspirin 300 mg, chewed, is also a key treatment therapy, particularly in the pre-hospital situation. It reduces the incidence of coronary re-occlusion following thrombolytic therapy and reduces the incidence of cardiac death. It should be given as soon as possible, so long as the casualty is not allergic to it or has an active peptic ulcer. If aspirin is chewed in the early stages of an acute MI, it is absorbed more quickly than if it is swallowed.

Pathogenesis

MI is commonly caused by the rupture of an atheromatous plaque in a coronary artery. Prior to rupture most of these plaques are not haemodynamically significant. Once the plaque ruptures the following events are triggered:

* haemorrhage into the plaque causing it to expand and restrict the lumen of the coronary artery

* smooth muscle contraction of the artery wall, further restricting the lumen

* thrombus formation on the surface of the ruptured plaque (platelet adhesion) leading to total obstruction of the coronary lumen.

Signs and symptoms

Typical signs and symptoms include:
* retrosternal chest pain; crushing in nature, often described as a tight 'band' or 'vice'; the pain is not relieved by GTN spray or rest

* pain can radiate into the neck, throat, jaw, back and down one or both arms (usually inner side of arm, under the axilla to the inner two fingers)

* sweating

* pallor

* cold and clammy skin

* nausea and vomiting
(Laird et al, 2004; Wyatt et al, 2005).

Sometimes the history can be unhelpful, e.g. an MI may develop without any significant chest pain. Sometimes it is difficult to distinguish between cardiac and indigestion pains

Treatment

- If MI suspected, alert the emergency services and stay with the casualty until they arrive (www.eguidelines.co.uk, February 2005); also telephone the casualty's own GP

- Help the casualty to adopt a relaxed position which reduces the myocardial workload: the patient will usually prefer to sit with the head and shoulders supported and knees bent (Fig. 9.1). A supine position can sometimes provoke or worsen the pain

- Reassure the casualty and encourage rest

- If the casualty is conscious give a full-dose (300 mg) aspirin tablet to chew slowly; do check first that there is no allergy to it. If aspirin is chewed in the early stages of an acute MI, it is absorbed more quickly than if it is swallowed

- If the casualty has a GTN spray or similar encourage its use as prescribed by the GP

- Closely monitor the casualty and be prepared to start BLS if it is required

Palpitations

Causes

Causes of palpitations include:
- ischaemic heart disease
- drugs
- tea/coffee
- alcohol
  (Jevon, 2002).

Treatment

- Sit the casualty down and ask if there have been previous palpitations
- Reassure the casualty

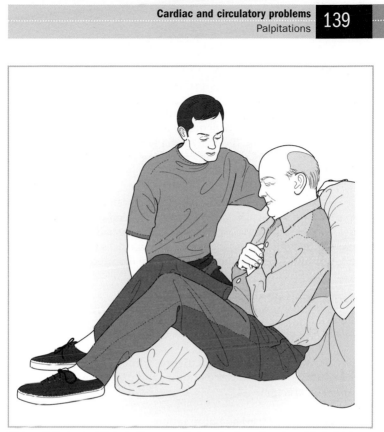

Figure 9.1 Acute MI: help the casualty to adopt a relaxed position which reduces the myocardial workload: they will usually prefer to sit with their head and shoulders supported and their knees bent

- Consider vagal stimulation: the most effective way of doing this is a Valsalva manoeuvre in the supine position; ask the casualty to cough or hold the nose and blow as if to pop the ears. Carotid sinus massage is another method of vagal stimulation, but can be dangerous, particularly in the elderly

- If the casualty is breathless, light-headed or has chest pain alert the emergency services; if the casualty has no symptoms but the palpitations do not settle, seek medical advice

Shock

Shock can be defined as 'a state of cardiovascular dysfunction resulting in a generalised inadequacy of tissue perfusion relative to metabolic requirements. Tissue hypoxia leads to progressive failure of cellular metabolism, eventually resulting in multiple organ dysfunction or death'.

If the casualty is in shock, the immediate provision of circulatory support is paramount. The prognosis will depend on the underlying cause, severity, duration of the shock, age of casualty and existence of any pre-existing illness. The emergency services must be alerted without delay, as oxygen and fluids may be required.

Classification of shock

There are four classifications of shock (Hinds & Watson, 1999):

Hypovolaemic shock: loss of circulating volume; causes include haemorrhaging, burns, severe vomiting and diarrhoea, and intestinal obstruction.

Cardiogenic shock: cardiac pump failure; causes include myocardial infarction, cardiac arrhythmias and myocarditis.

Distributive shock: abnormality of the peripheral circulation; causes include sepsis and anaphylaxis (anaphylaxis is covered in Chapter 7).

Obstructive shock: mechanical obstruction to cardiac output; causes include pulmonary embolism and cardiac tamponade.

Signs and symptoms

Signs and symptoms of shock include:
• cold and clammy skin

- pallor
- tachycardia
- tachypnoea
- yawning and sighing
- restlessness and agitation
  (British Red Cross, 2003).

(Signs and symptoms of anaphylactic shock are described on p. 101.)

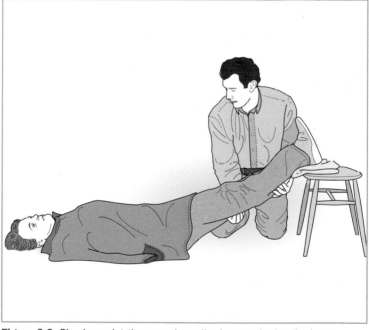

Figure 9.2 Shock: assist the casualty to lie down and raise the legs

Treatment

- Alert the emergency services
- Assist the casualty to lie down and raise the legs (British Red Cross, 2003) (Fig. 9.2)
- Reassure and keep the casualty warm
- Monitor the casualty
- Treat any obvious causes of the shock, e.g. apply pressure over external haemorrhaging

Conclusion

IHD is a leading cause of death in the Western world. Chest pain, a characteristic symptom of IHD, could indicate that the casualty is having an ACS. If this is the case, the emergency services should be alerted and the casualty transferred urgently to hospital for appropriate investigations and on-going care. This chapter has discussed the first aid treatment for cardiac and circulatory problems.

Neurological problems

Introduction

The nervous system, the most complex system in the body, can be affected by disease, injury or intoxication. If the functioning of the nervous system is compromised, the safety of the casualty can also be compromised, e.g. decreased conscious level can lead to the airway becoming compromised. It is therefore essential to ensure that a casualty with a problem affecting the nervous system is appropriately treated and managed.

The aim of this chapter is to understand the treatment of neurological problems.

Chapter objectives
At the end of the chapter the reader will be able to discuss the treatment of:

- **Fainting**

- **Headache**

- **Migraine**

- **Seizures**

- **Stroke**

- **Transient ischaemic attack**

- **Head injury**

Fainting

A faint can be defined as a brief loss of consciousness caused by a temporary reduction in blood flow to the brain. The medical term is syncope, derived from the Greek word 'to cut short'.
Approximately 30% of the population has experienced a fainting episode, many more have observed friends or colleagues have one.

Causes

The trigger is usually a sudden drop in blood pressure which has a number of causes including:
- warm environment
- prolonged standing
- sudden fright
- visual stimuli, e.g. sight of blood
- large meals
  (Brignole et al, 2001; Wyatt et al, 2005).

Signs and symptoms

Immediately prior to collapsing, the following signs and symptoms may be evident:
- sense of feeling unwell
- light-headedness or dizziness
- nausea
- sudden tiredness and yawning
- altered hearing
- blurred or tunnel vision
- pallor
- sudden collapse
  (Benditt & Goldstein, 2002; Wyatt et al, 2005).

If the casualty is unable to assume a supine position, e.g. being kept upright by bystanders, seizure-type twitching may occur (convulsive syncope).

Treatment

- If feeling faint, the casualty should be advised to lie down
- If the casualty starts to collapse, if possible support him to the floor (take care not to sustain an injury while doing so)
- Call out for help
- If necessary assess ABC to rule out cardiopulmonary arrest
- Kneel down and raise the casualty's legs above the level of the heart (Fig. 10.1)
- Get fresh air to the casualty: loosen any light clothing around the neck and chest, open a nearby window or door and request that any bystanders present do not crowd around the casualty
- Reassure the casualty
- Check for any injuries; if the casualty falls down during the faint, injuries such as bone fractures or a head injury could be sustained, particularly in the elderly
- If the casualty does not recover, place in the recovery position and call the emergency services; continually monitor ABC

Other considerations

- It is important to distinguish between an innocent 'simple faint' and a collapse due to a more sinister reason, e.g. a seizure or a cardiac event
- Note any neurological signs during the episode, or if not present at the time, obtain a detailed account of the episode from the casualty and from any bystanders who were present
- Cyanosis, tongue biting, saliva frothing at the mouth or incontinence suggest a generalised seizure
- Note the duration of the episode; if it is a simple faint, the casualty will recover very quickly, usually within 60 seconds

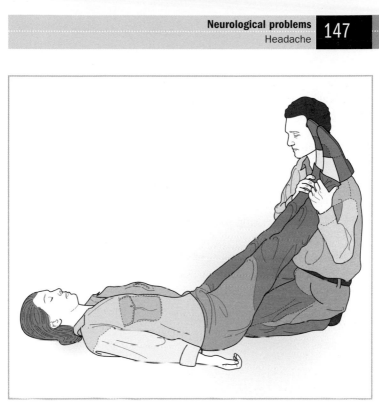

Figure 10.1 Fainting: raise the casualty's legs above the level of the heart

- Educate the casualty to recognise and avoid situations that could cause a faint

Headache

Causes

Causes of headaches include:
- tiredness
- tension
- influenza

- stress
- medications, e.g. nitrates
- excess alcohol.

A wide range of disorders can present with a headache. Sometimes a headache signifies a serious underlying pathology, e.g. subarachnoid haemorrhage, stroke, meningitis. It is important to ensure that these patients are not missed and that the emergency services are alerted.

Clinical features arousing particular concern are:
- very severe headache
- sudden severe headache
- photophobia
- altered level of consciousness
- associated neck rigidity
- developing rash
  (Wyatt et al, 2005).

Treatment

- Assist the casualty to sit or lie down in a quiet place
- Apply a cold compress to the casualty's head
- Ask casualty to take a simple analgesic drug if needed

When to alert the emergency services

Alert the emergency services if the headache is:
- of a sudden onset
- severe and incapacitating
- recurrent or persistent
- accompanied by neck rigidity
- associated with a head injury
- accompanied by a dazed feeling
  (British Red Cross, 2003).

Migraine

Migraine headaches affect approximately 6% of men and 18% of women and can last up to 72 hours. Prophylaxis may be indicated if the casualty is having two or more migraines per month. Advise the casualty to consult his GP.

Precipitants

Precipitants include:
- alcohol
- chocolate
- fatigue
- menstruation
- cheese
- shell-fish
- red wine
  (Wyatt et al, 2005).

Signs and symptoms

Typical signs and symptoms include:
- vision disturbance
- intense, throbbing headache, usually unilateral
- nausea and vomiting
- photophobia
  (Wyatt et al, 2005).

Treatment

- Assist the casualty to take analgesia or prescribed medication
- Advise the casualty to lie down, preferably in quiet, dark room and try to get some sleep

- Provide a bowl in case of vomiting
- Seek medical help if it is the casualty's first migraine, if vomiting is severe or if the casualty is concerned

Seizures

A seizure, sometimes referred to as a convulsion or fit, consists of involuntary muscle contractions. It is estimated that between 2 and 10% of the population will experience a seizure at some time in their life. There are over 40 different types of seizure and a person may have more than one type (Epilepsy Action, 2004).

Although seizures are rarely fatal, injuries are often sustained. Injuries that have been reported include fractures, burns, dislocations, concussion, and intracerebral haemorrhage. Dental injuries are quite common. Maintaining the casualty's safety during a seizure is a priority.

Causes

There are number of causes of seizures including:
- epilepsy (most common cause)
- head injury
- certain poisons, e.g. alcohol, ecstasy
- cerebral hypoxia
- cerebral hypoglycaemia.

Epilepsy

Epilepsy is a neurological disorder characterised by recurring seizures. An epileptic seizure is a brief, usually unprovoked, stereotyped disturbance of consciousness, behaviour, emotion, motor function or sensation resulting from abnormal cortical neuronal discharge. The outward manifestation of the seizure will depend on the part of the brain involved in the neuronal discharge.

The prevalence of active epilepsy is estimated to be between 430 and 1000 persons per 100 000 (Cockerell et al, 1994). In the UK, 440 000 (1:133) have epilepsy – making it the second most common neurological condition after migraine (Epilepsy Action, 2004). The majority of individuals (70–85%) with active epilepsy can satisfactorily control recurrent seizures with anti-epileptic drugs (Cilcot et al, 1999).

Sudden unexpected death in epilepsy is the principal cause of seizure-related death in people with chronic epilepsy, and has been estimated to account for approximately 500 deaths each year (National Institute for Clinical Excellence (NICE), 2002). Although it is not clear what causes these deaths, the most important risk factor is the occurrence of seizures – the more frequent the seizure, the higher the risk. A UK-wide audit of sudden unexpected death in epilepsy has found that 59% of child deaths and 39% of adult deaths could be potentially or probably avoidable (NICE, 2002).

Tonic–clonic seizure

A tonic–clonic seizure, formally termed grand mal fit, is typically characterised by:

- sudden loss of consciousness (often preceded by crying out) and collapse
- rigidity and arching of the back
- convulsive movements
- cyanosis around the mouth (due to irregular respirations)
- incontinence
- clenching of the jaw – saliva may appear at the mouth (could be blood-stained if the casualty has bitten the tongue or lip).

The convulsive movements should stop after a minute and consciousness should slowly return (the casualty may feel very tired and may fall into a deep sleep). The casualty may feel dazed and confused after the event (St John Ambulance, St Andrew's Ambulance, British Red Cross; Epilepsy Action, 2004).

The recommended first aid treatment for a tonic–clonic seizure is:

- protect the casualty from injury – ask bystanders to move away, make space around the casualty and remove any potentially dangerous objects, e.g. hot drinks, from the area if there is a risk of injury
- cushion the casualty's head – place something soft (e.g. a jumper or jacket) under the head or cup the head in your hands to prevent injury (Fig. 10.2)
- look for an epilepsy identity card or identity jewellery
- note the time to check how long the seizure is lasting
- once the seizure has stopped, check ABC. If the casualty is breathing place into the recovery position as soon as possible (if the casualty is not breathing, start resuscitation procedure – see Chapter 3)

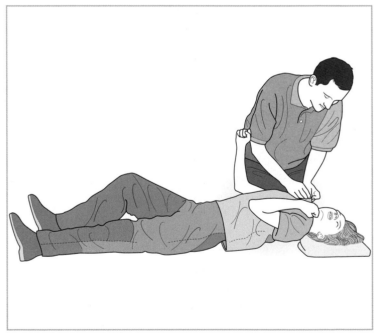

Figure 10.2 Tonic–clonic seizure: cushion the casualty's head – place something soft (e.g. a jumper or jacket) under the head or cup the head in your hands to prevent injury

- wipe away any saliva
- check for any injuries which may have been sustained
- calmly reassure the casualty
- stay with the casualty until recovery is complete (Epilepsy Action, 2004; National Society for Epilepsy, 2004).

The following is not recommended:
- restraining the casualty
- putting anything into the casualty's mouth
- trying to move the casualty, unless in danger
- giving the casualty something to eat or drink until recovery is complete
- attempting to arouse the casualty
  (Epilepsy Action, 2004; National Society for Epilepsy, 2004).

Seizures involving altered consciousness or behaviour

Simple partial seizures: twitching, numbness, sweating, dizziness or nausea; disturbances to hearing, vision, smell or taste; a strong sense of 'déjà vu'.

Complex partial seizures: plucking at clothes, smacking lips, swallowing repeatedly or wandering around; the casualty is unaware of his surroundings or of what he is doing.

Atonic seizures: sudden loss of muscle control causing the person to fall to the ground; recovery is quick.

Myoclonic seizures: brief forceful jerks which can affect the whole body or just part of it; the jerking could be severe enough to make the person fall.

Absence seizures (formally called petit mal fits): the casualty may appear to be daydreaming or switching off; he is momentarily unconscious and totally unaware of what is happening around him (Epilepsy Action, 2004).

The recommended first aid treatment of these types of seizures is:

- guide the casualty from danger
- look for an epilepsy identity card or identity jewellery
- stay with the casualty until recovery is complete
- calmly reassure the casualty
- explain anything that the casualty may have missed (Epilepsy Action, 2004).

The following is not recommended:
- restraining the casualty
- acting in a way that could frighten the casualty, e.g. making abrupt movements or shouting
- assuming the casualty is aware of what is happening, or what has happened
- giving the casualty something to eat or drink until recovery is complete
- attempting to arouse the casualty
  (Epilepsy Action, 2004).

If the casualty is not aware of his condition, advise him to consult his own GP as soon as possible (St John Ambulance, St Andrew's Ambulance, British Red Cross, 2002).

Status epilepticus

Status epilepticus can be defined as prolonged or recurrent tonic–clonic seizures lasting for 30 minutes or more. In pre-existing epilepsy, drug withdrawal or concurrent illness may be the cause; where there is no previous history of epilepsy, an acute cerebral event is usually the cause. Generalised tonic–clonic epilepsy, a medical emergency, is associated with significant morbidity and mortality if not treated promptly.

The aim of treatment is to halt seizures and prevent irreversible cerebral, systemic, metabolic, autonomic and cardiovascular changes. It is clearly important to alert the emergency services immediately and, while awaiting their arrival, maintain the safety of the casualty (see above for tonic–clonic seizures).

When to call the emergency services
....

Epilepsy Action (2004) recommends that the emergency services
should be contacted if:

- it is the casualty's first seizure
- the seizure continues for more than 5 minutes
- one tonic–clonic seizure follows another without the casualty regaining
  consciousness between seizures (status epilepticus)
- the casualty is injured during the seizure
- the casualty requires urgent medical attention.

What to observe for during a seizure
....

'A clear history from the casualty and an eyewitness to the attack
gives the most important diagnostic information, and should be the
mainstay of diagnosis' (SIGN, 2003). So as well as maintaining the
casualty's safety, observe the casualty during the seizure. The
following information can help with diagnosis and confirming
what type of seizure the casualty is having.

- Where was the casualty and what was he doing prior to the seizure?
- Any mood change, e.g. excitement, anger or anxiety?
- Unusual sensations, e.g. odd smell or taste?
- Any prior warning?
- Loss of consciousness or confusion?
- Any colour change, e.g. pallor, cyanosis? If so where, e.g. face, lips, hand?
- Altered respiratory pattern, e.g. dyspnoea, noisy respirations?
- Which part of the body affected by the seizure?
- Incontinence?
- Tongue biting?
- Did the casualty do anything unusual, e.g. mumble, wander about or
  fumble with his clothing?
- How long did the seizure last?

- How was the casualty following the seizure? Did the casualty need to sleep and if so, for how long?
- How long before the casualty can perform normal activities again? (National Society of Epilepsy, 2004).

Stroke

A stroke can be defined as a disruption in the blood supply to a region of the brain resulting in neurological impairment. Each year over 130 000 people in England and Wales suffer a stroke; about 10 000 of these are under retirement age (Office for National Statistics, 1991) and most occur at home. Annually there are close to 60 000 deaths due to stroke each year in England and Wales (Office for National Statistics, 1998).

Although the incidence of strokes and mortality from strokes is falling in most countries, the gain achieved by prevention has been counterbalanced by a rise in the ageing (high risk) population.

Strokes can be classified into two major categories, ischaemic and haemorrhagic. Cerebral ischaemia causes 85% of all strokes, usually due to an embolism or thrombosis.

Stroke is a medical emergency that requires hospital care. Successful acute stroke intervention depends on early hospital presentation. Hospital admission delay is a main limiting factor for effective thrombolytic therapy in stroke patients.

Signs and symptoms

Signs and symptoms of a stroke are very similar to a TIA. However, they will persist longer than 24 hours and could include:
- unilateral paralysis: weakness or heaviness, usually involving one side of the body
- unilateral numbness: sensory loss, numbness or abnormal sensation, usually involving one side of the body

- language disturbance: aphasia or slurred speech
- monocular blindness: partial visual loss in one eye
- vertigo: sense of spinning, even at rest
- ataxia: poor balance or staggering
  (American Heart Association & ILCOR, 2000).

Treatment

- Assess ABC
- Alert the emergency services
- If conscious, ensure the casualty's head and shoulders are supported in a slightly raised position, to help protect the airway
- Tilt the casualty's head towards the weaker side, thus allowing secretions etc to drain out; wipe the mouth with a flannel or similar (Fig. 10.3)

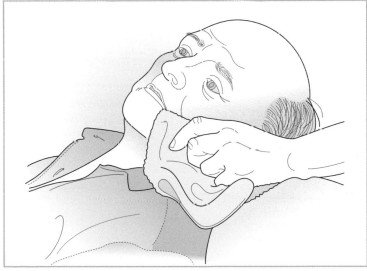

Figure 10.3 Stroke: ensure the casualty's head and shoulders are supported in a slightly raised position, to help protect the airway and tilt the head towards the weaker side, thus allowing secretions etc to drain out

- Ensure the casualty's airway remains patent: aspiration of gastric contents or secretions is a serious complication associated with considerable morbidity and mortality
- Do not give the casualty anything to eat or drink
- Regularly monitor vital signs, particularly the patency of the airway
- If unconscious, place the casualty in the recovery position

Transient ischaemic attack

A transient ischaemic attack (TIA) can be defined as an episode of transient focal neurological deficit lasting less than 24 hours. The cause is either thrombosis or embolism. A TIA is usually of a short duration, rarely persisting for more than 5 minutes, but symptoms may last up to 24 hours. There are between 30 000 and 40 000 TIAs every year in the UK (Stroke Assocation, 2005). A TIA is often referred to as a mini-stroke.

Following a TIA, 5% within 48 hours and up to 50% within 5 years will have a stroke (Wyatt et al, 2004). A TIA should never be ignored – seek urgent medical attention.

Signs and symptoms

- Numbness
- Weakness of one part of the body
- Headache
- Uncoordinated speech
- Limited visual field
- Dizziness, nausea or deafness
  (Stroke Association, 2005).

Treatment

Most TIAs last only minutes. Therefore only minimal treatment will be required:

- maintain the casualty's safety; assess ABC
- reassure the casualty
- encourage to seek urgent medical help as further investigation and follow-up will be needed; it may be necessary to alert the emergency services.

Head injury

Head injury is very common. Approximately 10% of patients presenting to A & E have suffered a head injury, though most attenders only have a mild injury. However, all head injuries are potentially serious because they can damage the brain and surrounding blood vessels. Although the skull protects the brain, it also provides an enclosed space in which the brain can be shaken and damaged and where there is little room for bleeding and swelling following an injury.

Concussion, cerebral compression and a fractured skull can complicate a head injury. Practically, it is important to be able to recognise each one (Table 10.1). Cerebral compression and a fractured skull require the casualty to be urgently transferred to hospital.

History

Take a history of the incident, though this will be difficult if the casualty suffered a period of unconsciousness and/or has amnesia. Use other sources of information, e.g. relatives, friends, work colleagues, bystanders etc. Information that will be very helpful includes:

- mechanism of injury
- time of injury
- whether the casualty sustained an alteration in mental status or unconsciousness
  (American Heart Association, 2000).

Table 10.1 Recognition of concussion, cerebral compression and a fractured skull

Concussion	Cerebral compression	Skull fracture
Brief period of impaired consciousness following a blow to the head	Deteriorating level of response – may progress to unconsciousness	Wound or bruise on the head
There may also be:	There may also be:	Soft area or depression on the scalp
Dizziness or nausea on recovery	History of recent head injury	Bruising/swelling behind one ear
Loss of memory of any events that occurred at the time of, or immediately preceding, the injury	Intense headache	Bruising around one or both eyes
Mild, generalised headache	Noisy breathing, becoming slow	Loss of clear fluid or watery blood from the nose or an ear
	Slow, yet full and strong, pulse	Blood in the white of the eye
	Unequal pupil size	Distortion or lack of symmetry of head or face
	Weakness and/or paralysis down one side of the face and/or body	Deteriorating level of response – may progress to unconsciousness
	High temperature; flushed face	
	Drowsiness	
	Noticeable change in personality or behaviour, such as irritability	

Source: St John Ambulance, 2002

Causes

Causes of head injury include:
- road traffic accident
- fall
- assault

- sport
- electrocution/lightning strike.

When to suspect a head injury

Suspect a head injury if the casualty:
- fell from a height greater than his own
- was unconscious when found
- sustained a blunt force injury
- sustained a high-impact sports injury
- sustained an injury caused by diving, electrocution, a lightning strike or was wearing a protective helmet that was inadequate or broken (American Heart Association, 2000).

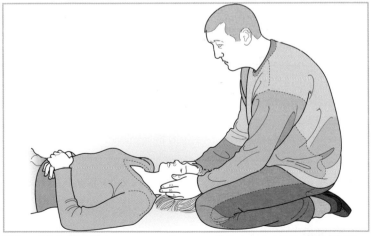

Figure 10.4 Head injury: assume the casualty has a cervical spine injury: maintain the head in the neutral position, with the head, neck and spine aligned

Treatment

- Assume the casualty has a cervical spine injury: maintain the head in the neutral position, with the head, neck and spine aligned (Fig. 10.4)
- If the airway is compromised, use jaw thrust to open it
- If the casualty is breathing, try to leave him in the position he has been found
- Monitor the casualty's vital signs
- Check the level of consciousness using AVPU
- Ensure the emergency services have been alerted
- Apply direct pressure to control any bleeding from the scalp

When to refer to hospital

- Period of impaired consciousness
- Amnesia, either of the incident or subsequent events
- Vomiting, seizures, severe and persistent headaches
- Evidence of skull fracture – yellowish, blood-stained fluid discharge from the ear or nose
- Significant scalp injury
- Worrying mechanism of injury, e.g. penetrating or high velocity injury
- Uncertainty of diagnosis
- Medical co-morbidity, e.g. anti-coagulant therapy
- Alcohol abuse
- Adverse social conditions, e.g. casualty living alone
  (Wyatt et al, 2004)

NICE has issued guidelines on head injury (2003). Boxes 10.1 and 10.2 detail some helpful advice.

Concussion

Concussion is when the brain is 'shaken' by a blow to the head. It produces an alteration in mental status, particularly confusion and

> **Box 10.1** Signs that an ambulance should be called
>
> · Unconsciousness, or lack of full consciousness (for example, problems keeping eyes open)
> · Problems understanding, speaking, reading or writing
> · Loss of feeling in part of the body
> · Problems balancing or walking
> · General weakness
> · Any changes in eyesight
> · Any clear fluid running from ears or nose
> · A black eye with no associated damage around the eye
> · Bleeding from one or both ears
> · New deafness in one or both ears
> · Bruising behind one or both ears
> · Any evidence of scalp or skull damage, especially when the skull has been penetrated
> · A forceful blow to the head at speed (e.g. a pedestrian struck by a car, a car or bicycle crash, a diving accident, a fall of 1 metre or more (less in the case of a child or baby), or a fall down more than five stairs (less in the case of a child or baby))
> · Any convulsions or having a fit

amnesia, and may or may not include loss of consciousness. This disturbance in consciousness is transient.

Treatment for concussion is:
• help the casualty to sit or lie down
• reassure casualty
• monitor conscious level
• on recovery, ensure that the casualty stays with a responsible person for a few hours
• advise the casualty to seek medical help if he later develops headache, nausea, vomiting or excessive sleepiness.

If the casualty does not fully recover, or if he deteriorates after an initial recovery, alert the emergency services

> **Box 10.2** Signs that the person should go or be taken to an A & E department straightaway (an ambulance should be called if this can't be done safely)
>
> - Any loss of consciousness (being 'knocked out') from which the person has now recovered
> - Any problems with memory
> - A headache that won't go away
> - Any vomiting or sickness
> - Previous brain surgery
> - A history of bleeding problems or taking medicine (e.g. warfarin) that may cause bleeding problems
> - Age 65 years or more
> - Irritability or altered behaviour such as being easily distracted, not themselves, no concentration, or no interest in things around them, particularly in infants and young children (younger than 5 years)
> - The person is drunk or has taken drugs
> - Suspicion that the injury was caused intentionally by the person himself or herself, or by someone else

NB The injured person should see his GP if he or the person looking after him has any worries concerning the head injury, even if he doesn't have any of the signs listed in Boxes 10.1 and 10.2, or if there is nobody to look after him at home.

Conclusion

The nervous system can be affected by disease, injury or intoxication. Problems affecting the nervous system can be life-threatening. If the functioning of the nervous system is compromised, the safety of the casualty can also be compromised, particularly if the casualty's conscious level is altered. In this chapter problems affecting the nervous system have been discussed.

Diabetic emergencies

Diabetic emergencies

Introduction

In the UK, approximately 3% of the population has diabetes (Watkins, 2003). It can be classified as Type 1 or Type 2.

- Type 1 diabetes (previously insulin-dependent diabetes) is complete insulin deficiency due to destruction of B-cells in the islets of Langerhans in the pancreas. Peak incidence is in the 10–12 years age group; usually presents in the <40 year age group. It is treated by insulin injections, and diet and regular exercise is recommended.

- Type 2 diabetes (previously non-insulin-dependent diabetes) ranges from predominant insulin resistance associated with relative insulin deficiency to predominant insulin secretory defect with insulin resistance; usually idiopathic, it is most commonly seen in the 50–70 years age group. It is treated by diet and exercise alone or by diet, exercise and medication or by diet, exercise and insulin.

Normal plasma glucose levels range from 3.6 to 5.8 mmol/l. Both hypoglycaemia and hyperglycaemia, which can both complicate diabetes, can be life-threatening.

The aim of this chapter is to understand the first aid treatment of diabetic emergencies.

Chapter objectives
At the end of the chapter the reader will be able to:

- **Discuss the treatment of hypoglycaemia**

- **Discuss the treatment of hyperglycaemia**

Hypoglycaemia

Hypoglycaemia can be defined as a blood glucose level <4 mmol/l. It is difficult to estimate the true incidence of hypoglycaemic episodes, as most are treated successfully at home and some, particularly those occurring at night, may not be recognised.

Repeated episodes of hypoglycaemia can cause extreme emotional distress, even when the episodes are relatively mild. Education is the key to prevent recurrent or severe hypoglycaemia.

Causes

Common causes of hypoglycaemia include:
- too much insulin
- delayed or missed meal or snack
- not enough food, especially carbohydrate
- unplanned or strenuous exercise
- alcohol consumption without food
- idiopathic
  (Diabetes UK, 2002).

Alcohol intake can lead to hypoglycaemia several hours later; the effects of alcohol may also mask hypoglycaemic symptoms. Medical causes of hypoglycaemia include liver failure, Addison's disease and pituitary insufficiency.

Signs and symptoms

The signs and symptoms vary from person to person, though they are often constant for an individual. Individuals may recognise different symptoms and these may change as the duration of diabetes increases. Signs and symptoms of hypoglycaemia include:
- shaking
- sweating

- hunger
- pins and needles in the lips and tongue
- altered level of consciousness
- tachycardia
- nausea and vomiting.

Generally, the casualty can recognise the development of hypoglycaemia, though this may not always be the case. In addition, recurrent hypoglycaemic episodes can lead to diminished casualty awareness of impending hypoglycaemia.

Treatment for mild hypoglycaemia

- Look for a MedicAlert bracelet/chain
- If the casualty's conscious level allows him safely to eat and drink, offer the simplest available food that contains carbohydrate that can be quickly absorbed, e.g. sugary foods:
  - glass of Lucozade or coke (not diet drinks)
  - glass of fruit juice
  - five sweets, e.g. barley sugar
  - three or more glucose tablets
    (Diabetes UK, 2002)
- Monitor the casualty's response and conscious level
- If the casualty has a blood glucose testing kit, assist in measuring the blood glucose level – this is the only way to establish whether the casualty does have hypoglycaemia
- Try to establish the possible cause of the hypoglycaemia
- Encourage the casualty to see his GP if necessary

Then, to prevent a repeat hypoglycaemic episode, offer the casualty food containing starchy carbohydrates (absorbed more slowly), e.g. a sandwich, fruit, bowl of cereal or biscuits and milk.

Treatment for severe hypoglycaemia

- If the casualty is unconscious place in the recovery position and monitor vital signs
- Look for a MedicAlert bracelet/chain
- Alert the emergency services
- If available, administer Hypostop (a dextrose gel, rapidly absorbed via the buccal mucosa)

Glucagon

Glucagon, a hormone produced by the A-cells of the islets in the pancreas, increases the blood glucose level by mobilising glycogen stores in the liver. The majority of people with Type 1 diabetes lose their glucagon response to hypoglycaemia within 5 years of diagnosis.

Glucagon 1 mg I/M is very effective at reversing hypoglycaemia (Watkins, 2003). It is particularly useful for a bystander of a severely hypoglycaemic casualty who is unable to take oral glucose, and can be administered by family members, nurses or doctors.

Risks for the casualty

If there is a deterioration in the casualty's conscious level, then the airway can become compromised. Ensure that the casualty's airway remains patent. If the casualty is unconscious, place in the recovery position.

Although the risks of hazard from hypoglycaemia are small, a prolonged severe hypoglycaemic episode can cause moderate to severe neuropsychological impairments. Hypoglycaemia can cause an acute cerebral injury, causing hemiplegia.

Education

Education is the key to preventing recurrent or severe hypoglycaemia. In particular, casualty education should emphasise the role of blood glucose monitoring in relation to driving, and highlight the potential deterioration in driving performance when blood glucose falls below 4.0 mmol/l (Graveling & Warren, 2004).

If the casualty is unconscious place in recovery position, with particular attention to maintaining a clear airway.

Hyperglycaemia

Hyperglycaemia is an abnormally high blood sugar level. Undiagnosed diabetics in the younger age group often present with hyperglycaemia (due to lack of insulin) and diabetic ketoacidosis (DKA). The body's inability to utilise the circulating glucose leads to the metabolism of fat, resulting in the release of ketones and metabolic acidosis (DKA) (Jones et al, 2003). The casualty will require treatment in hospital.

Signs and symptoms

Signs and symptoms of hyperglycaemia include:
- hyperventilation
- tachycardia
- extreme thirst
- polydipsia
- polyuria
- altered conscious level
  (Wyatt et al, 2005).

Treatment

- If casualty is unconscious place in recovery position
- Look for a MedicAlert bracelet/chain
- Monitor casualty's vital signs
- Alert the emergency services

In the first aid setting, it can be difficult to distinguish between hypoglycaemia and hyperglycaemia: if the casualty is a known diabetic and is unwell, offer a sugary drink: this will help to correct hypoglycaemia, but will do little harm if it is actually hyperglycaemia (British Red Cross, 2003)

Conclusion

Diabetes can be classified as Type 1 diabetes (complete insulin deficiency) and Type 2 diabetes (ranges from predominant insulin resistance associated with relative insulin deficiency to predominant insulin secretory defect with insulin resistance). Hypoglycaemia and hyperglycaemia can be life-threatening and this chapter has outlined the first aid treatment for both.

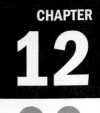

Extremes in body temperature

Introduction

The thermoregulatory centre in the hypothalamus maintains body temperature between 36 and 37°C. The body can only function effectively within a narrow temperature range; severe hypothermia or hyperthermia can lead to life-threatening complications.

Pyrexia in response to infection is a protective mechanism, inhibiting bacterial and viral growth, promoting immunity and phagocytosis and through hypermetabolism encouraging tissue repair. Mild pyrexia is therefore generally not treated.

The aim of this chapter is to understand the principles of first aid management of extremes in body temperature.

Chapter objectives
At the end of the chapter the reader will be able to:

- **Discuss the treatment for hypothermia**

- **Describe the treatment for frostbite**

- **Outline the treatment for sunburn**

- **Discuss the treatment for heat exhaustion**

- **Discuss the treatment for heat stroke**

Hypothermia

Hypothermia is defined as a core temperature of <35°C. It can be classified as:

- mild hypothermia (32–35°C)
- moderate hypothermia (30–32°C)
- severe hypothermia (<30°C)
  (Wyatt et al, 2005).

Risk factors

Hypothermia can occur if the body loses too much heat or is unable to maintain its normothermic state. Risk factors for hypothermia include:

- increased age (impaired thermoregulation, reduced metabolism)
- altered conscious level
- drugs
- alcohol
- exposure (inadequate warm clothing, inadequate heating, following submersion)
- endocrine (hypoglycaemia, hypothyroidism)
- malnutrition
- autonomic neuropathy (Parkinson's disease, diabetes mellitus)
  (Ramrakha & Moore, 2004).

Signs and symptoms

Signs and symptoms of hypothermia can vary depending on its severity. Common findings include:

- deterioration in conscious level
- pallor
- cold skin
- slurred and incomprehensible speech

- lethargy
- weak pulse.

Severe hypothermia can mimic death

Treatment

- If possible, prevent further heat loss, e.g. remove wet clothes and replace with dry ones; if outdoors use warm, dry clothing from bystanders
- Offer a warm drink
- If the casualty is young and fit and can get into a bath unaided, consider this method of rewarming, ensuring the water is approximately 40°C
- For additional warmth, cover the casualty's head
- If outdoors, ensure the casualty is sheltered (if possible) and insulated from the cold ground
- Seek medical help or arrange transfer to hospital as appropriate
- Regularly monitor the casualty's vital signs
- Keep movement of the casualty to a minimum, and be gentle; casualty movement can produce life-threatening cardiac arrhythmias

Do not:
- Offer the casualty alcohol
- Advise the casualty to exercise
- Apply direct heat, e.g. hot water bottles or sitting next to a radiator
- Re-warm the casualty too quickly (peripheral vasodilation can induce hypotension and further drop core temperature).

Frostbite

Frostbite is caused by the freezing of peripheral tissues, leading to tissue necrosis. It usually affects the fingers and toes and the casualty may also be hypothermic. Shelter, insulation and external warmth are necessary in prevention and thawing of frozen parts.

Risk factors

- Sub-zero temperatures, particularly when exposure to wind results in wind chill
- Poor tissue perfusion, e.g. in hypovolaemic shock

Signs and symptoms

- Pins and needles and loss of sensation in affected area
- Initially pallor, then mottled and cyanosed; if gangrene develops, the skin usually turns black

Treatment

- If possible, help the casualty to a warm environment
- Gently remove constricting objects/clothing, e.g. rings, gloves, boots
- Attempt to warm the affected part, e.g. with your hands (do not rub) or place it in the casualty's armpit
- Cover affected part with a dressing/bandage to protect it; mechanical injury must be avoided if tissue loss is to be minimised
- Arrange transfer to hospital

Do not:
- Rub the affected part
- Apply direct heat, e.g. hot water bottle
- Try to thaw affected part if there is a possibility of it re-freezing
- Allow the casualty to smoke
  (St John Ambulance, 2002).

Sunburn

Sunburn is be caused by too much exposure to the sun (even on a cloudy day), sunbeds and sun lamps. Factors that increase the risk of sunburn include high altitudes, reflective surfaces, e.g. snow and sand, and sweating. Sunburn can lead to heat exhaustion and heat stroke.

Signs and symptoms

Signs and symptoms of sunburn include:
- red skin
- pain in the affected area
- skin blisters (later).

Treatment

- Help the casualty to a cool area, out of the sun
- Offer the casualty frequent small sips of cold water as there may be dehydration
- Remove clothing
- Cool the skin surface: tepid sponging or soak affected area in a cold bath for 10 minutes
- For mild sunburn: apply calamine lotion; for severe sunburn seek medical help
- Monitor the casualty's vital signs

Heat exhaustion

Heat exhaustion is caused by an abnormal loss of sodium and water due to excessive sweating. It can occur following excessive exercise and in hot weather. If untreated, heat stroke can develop which can prove fatal.

Signs and symptoms

Signs and symptoms of heat exhaustion include:
* temperature <40°C
* normal mental function
* weakness and fatigue
* headache
* nausea and vomiting
  (Wyatt et al, 2005).

Treatment

* Help the casualty to lie down in a cool environment and raise the legs to facilitate cerebral perfusion
* Offer casualty plenty of cool water
* Remove clothing and apply surface cooling, e.g. fan, tepid sponge
* Closely monitor the casualty's core temperature to avoid overshoot hypothermia and rebound hyperthermia
* If the casualty recovers, ensure a GP is consulted; if not alert the emergency services

Heat stroke

Heat stroke or severe hyperthermia is a temperature >40°C. It can be caused by 'ecstasy', prolonged hot weather, vigorous activity and certain drugs (malignant hyperthermia).

Heat stroke can develop if the symptoms of heat exhaustion are not recognised and treated. It can cause organ failure, cerebral damage and death. It carries a mortality risk of 10%. During a heat wave in London in 2003, deaths in the >75 years age group increased by 60%; in the same year, a heat wave in Northern France resulted in

15 000 excess deaths, mostly among the elderly population
(Department of Health, 2005a).

Risk factors

Those at particularly at risk of heat stroke include:
- older people, especially those >75 years of age and /or living on their
  own or in a care home
- people with mental health problems or dementia
- people who rely on others to manage normal daily activities
- people who are bed-bound
- infants and children
  (Department of Health, 2005).

In addition, environments such as accommodation in top floor flats,
lack of air conditioning and work places producing heat, e.g.
foundries and bakeries, can exacerbate the risk of extreme heat.

Signs and symptoms

Signs and symptoms of heat stroke include:
- tachypnoea
- tachycardia
- altered mental status, e.g. confusion
- temperature >40°C.

Treatment

- Alert the emergency services
- Continue active cooling until the core temperature is <39°C: remove
  clothing, ensure a cool environment and apply surface cooling, e.g. fan,
  tepid sponge; if possible apply 'tepid sponging' using a spray water
  device

- Monitor the casualty's vital signs
- Closely monitor the casualty's core temperature to avoid overshoot hypothermia and rebound hyperthermia

Conclusion

The human body can only function effectively within a narrow temperature range; severe hypothermia or hyperthermia can lead to life-threatening complications. This chapter has outlined the principles of first aid management of extremes in temperature.

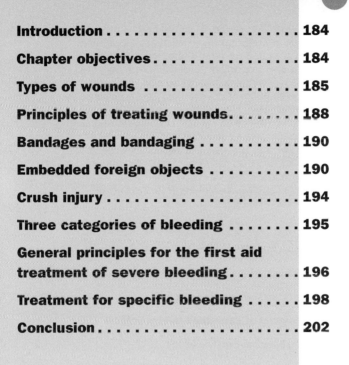

CHAPTER 13

Wounds and bleeding

Introduction

Wounds can be classified as being either open wounds, e.g. abrasion, puncture wound, or closed wounds, e.g. bruise. Wounds and bleeding can be life-threatening. When providing first aid, it is important to be able to recognise which wounds can be managed at home and which will require urgent medical attention. Wounds can be caused by a number of mechanisms; the treatment and management of wounds is often determined by the mechanism of injury.

When providing first aid for wounds and bleeding, it is important to ensure that the risk of infection is minimised, both to the rescuer and the casualty. If possible, sterile gloves should be worn.

The aim of this chapter is to understand the first aid treatment of wounds and bleeding.

Chapter objectives
At the end of the chapter the reader will be able to:

- **List the types of wounds**

- **Discuss the principles of treating wounds**

- **Outline the treatment of embedded foreign objects**

- **Discuss the treatment of crush injuries**

- **Discuss the treatment of an amputated limb or digit**

- **Outline the three categories of bleeding**

- **Discuss the general principles for the first aid treatment of severe bleeding**

- **Discuss the treatment for specific types of bleeding**

Wounds and bleeding
Types of wounds
185

Types of wounds

Wounds manifest in a variety of ways. All require assessment and treatment and all need to be treated as a unique occurrence. Tetanus needs to be considered and vaccination given if necessary.

Wounds may be categorised as follows.

Abrasion (graze)

An abrasion, commonly referred to as a graze, is a superficial injury manifesting from the ripping of skin. It can be caused by a friction burn or gravel rash. Tags of skin may be evident at one end of the abrasion, indicating the edge of skin last in contact with the abrading surface. Such wounds are often contaminated with foreign bodies and infection can result.

Incised wound

An incised wound (Fig. 13.1) is a cut caused by a sharp object, e.g. knife, broken glass. Vascular damage may occur resulting in profuse bleeding. Structural damage to tendons or nerves may be complicating factors.

Laceration

A laceration is tearing or ripping of the skin; it may be superficial or may involve deeper structures. It may be caused by barbed wire, jagged metal or broken glass. Unlike most incised wounds, haemorrhage generally tends to be less profuse, but soft tissue damage adjacent to the laceration can be significant and the risk of infection is high.

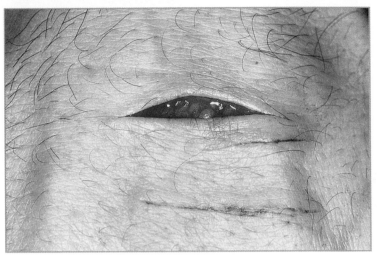

Figure 13.1 Incised wound. Reproduced with permission from O'Shea, Principles & Practice of Trauma Nursing, Elsevier Ltd

Puncture wound

A puncture wound is normally caused by a sharp object. It can manifest in a number of ways, not all being obvious. Insect, plant or marine life can all cause puncture wounds. Equally, man-made punctures can manifest in the form of penetrating wounds from knives or other sharp objects or from accidental impalement.

Stab wound

A stab wound is inherently a puncture wound, yet somewhat surgical in nature, due to it being caused by knives or other bladed instruments. These wounds may be significant and life-threatening. Internal and external haemorrhage may be profuse.

Wounds and bleeding
Types of wounds
187

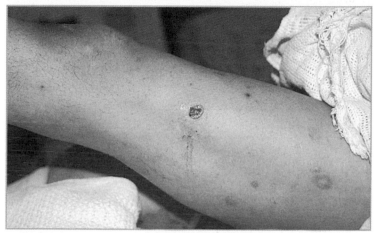

Figure 13.2 Gunshot wound. Reproduced with permission from O'Shea, Principles & Practice of Trauma Nursing, Elsevier Ltd

Gunshot wound

A gunshot wound (Fig. 13.2) is caused by a bullet or missile. The severity is dependent upon the velocity of the weapon used. Entry and exit wounds are common, although the projectile may remain in situ. Usually manifest in a small entry and large exit wound.

Bruise

A bruise, sometimes referred to as a contusion, is caused by a blunt injury to blood vessels within the tissues, resulting in tender swelling and discoloration.

The site of the bruise will change in colour as the bruise develops. At its peak the bruise will be blue/black in nature, eventually fading to show a yellow pigment by about day five. This manifestation is the bilirubin leaking from the damaged red blood cells and is part of the bruise's normal pathology. Extensive bruising can last for several weeks.

The normal course of a bruise is to present with significant pain and lack of power and movement. Treatment consists of a cold compress, rest and elevation.

Degloving injury

A degloving injury, normally associated with major trauma, results from a parallel force being applied to the skin, tearing away layers of tissue and usually exposing deeper anatomical structures.

Principles of treating wounds

The treatment for wounds usually depends on the mechanism of injury and the type of wound caused, e.g. laceration, puncture wound etc. Whether there is tissue loss or not will also influence wound treatment.

The risk of infection, especially tetanus, is of particular concern. As the skin is broken, all wounds are effectively contaminated and infection is possible. Wounds more than 6 hours old are more likely to become infected.

Wound assessment

When assessing a wound the following should be established:
- mechanism of injury – in particular, is internal injury likely?
- time of injury
- place of injury, e.g. in the garden, i.e. tetanus risk
- tetanus status of the casualty
- location of the wound
- circulation problems distal to the wound

- extent of likely damage
- in the case of a burn/scald – surface area and depth of skin affected
- amount of bleeding and what type
- presence of foreign body
  (Jones et al, 2003).

Anti-tetanus prophylaxis

The need for anti-tetanus prophylaxis should also be considered. There are approximately 30–40 tetanus cases in the UK each year; *Clostridium tetani* spores are commonly found in soil and animal faeces. Anti-tetanus prophylaxis will depend upon the tetanus status of the casualty and whether the wound is 'clean' or 'tetanus-prone', e.g. puncture wound, animal bite.

Cleaning a wound

If necessary, wash the wound under running tap water; tap water does not contain pathogenic bacteria and is often used in A & E departments to clean acute traumatic wounds; if the tap water is unsuitable for drinking, boil and then cool the water or use bottled drinking water. If possible remove foreign bodies (unless embedded in a deep wound). Dry the wound and apply a dressing (sterile if possible).

Dressings

Applying a dressing will help to keep the wound dry and will provide some degree of protection. There are many different types of wound dressings currently available. Some important points to consider when using a dressing:

- ensure the dressing is large enough to fit comfortably cover the wound
- use a sterile dressing if possible; if not available, a clean non-fluffy dressing will suffice
- when applying the dressing, ensure to handle it using its edges

- use adhesive dressing for small cuts and grazes
- if applying a plaster always check first that the casualty does not have an allergy to it.

Bandages and bandaging

Bandages can be used to secure dressings, control bleeding, immobilise and support limbs and reduce swelling. The key principles of bandaging are discussed in Chapter 20.

Cold compress

The application of a cold compress can help to reduce swelling and relieve pain. It can be particularly helpful for treating bruising and sprains. There are two methods of applying a cold press: a cold pad or an ice pack.

Cold pad

- Soak a pad (towel, flannel or similar) in cold water; then wring it out
- Apply the pad firmly over the injury
- Regularly re-soak the pad in cold water to keep it cold

Ice pack

- Partly fill a plastic bag with ice cubes and then seal it (a bag of frozen vegetables will suffice)
- Wrap it up in a dry cloth or towel
- Apply the pad firmly over the injury
- Replace the bag as required

Do not apply ice directly onto the skin, as it may burn it

Embedded foreign objects

Embedded foreign objects can be very painful and can cause infection. Only remove them if it is easy to do so; otherwise seek medical help.

*Seek urgent medical help for embedded large foreign objects,
particularly those in the chest and abdomen*

Splinter

If the casualty has a small splinter, e.g. of wood, glass or metal, it
may be possible to remove it using a pair of tweezers:

- sterilise a pair of tweezers, e.g. place in boiling water for a few seconds
  and then let them cool

- gently squeeze the skin either side of the splinter; hopefully the splinter
  will then be protruding out from the skin

- using the tweezers, grasp the splinter and pull it out at the angle it went
  in (Fig. 13.3)

- carefully squeeze the wound to encourage slight bleeding to flush out
  any remaining dirt

- clean and dry the area and apply adhesive dressing if necessary.

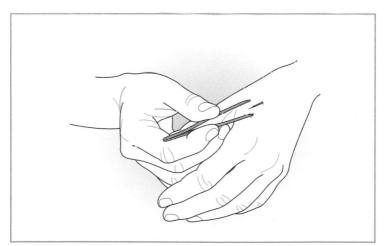

Figure 13.3 Removal of a splinter: using the tweezers, grasp the splinter
and pull it out at the angle it went in

Embedded fish-hook

A fish-hook can easily become embedded in the skin, usually a finger. The barb makes it very difficult to remove, as it prevents the hook from being withdrawn.

Medical help readily available

- Sever the fishing line as close to the hook as possible
- Place pads of gauze around the hook sufficient enough to be able to bandage over the hook without applying pressure on it
- Ensure the casualty seeks medical attention

Medical help not readily available

- Sever the fishing line as close to the hook as possible
- Cut the barb using a pair of pliers or wire cutters (ideally wear eye protection and ask casualty to look away); if the barb is not visible, push it quickly and firmly until it emerges, cut it off, then withdraw it
- Grasping the eye of the hook, gently withdraw it
- Clean wound and apply dressing
- Check tetanus status of the casualty and seek medical advice if necessary

Large embedded object

A large embedded object in a wound should be left in situ, as further damage may be caused, particularly if it is in the chest or abdomen (the object may have pierced a blood vessel and, while it remains in the wound, may act as a 'plug' and prevent bleeding). First aid treatment:

- if there is bleeding from around the embedded object, apply pressure around it; do not apply pressure to the actual object
- place pads of gauze around the object sufficient enough to be able to bandage over it without applying pressure on it (Fig. 13.4)
- elevate the affected limb if appropriate
- seek medical help.

Wounds and bleeding
Embedded foreign objects
193

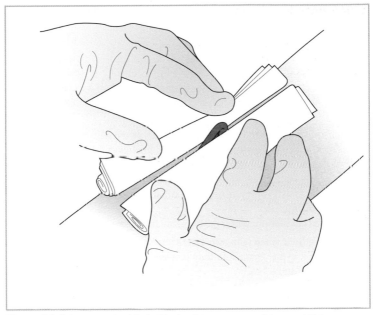

Figure 13.4 Large embedded object: place gauze pads around the embedded object sufficiently high enough to be able to bandage over it without applying pressure on it

Impalement

If the casualty has an impalement injury, e.g. after falling onto railings, do not attempt lifting off the object because this may worsen any internal injuries. Great care is needed to ensure that the injury is not worsened by the rescuer's desire to help.

First aid treatment:
- alert the emergency services and provide accurate details of the situation: this is a specialist circumstance and requires the involvement of the Fire & Rescue Service or Ambulance Service SCAT (Special Casualty Access Team)

- while awaiting the arrival of the emergency services, if possible support the casualty.

Do not remove impaled objects

Crush injury

A crush injury is when tissue is squashed. It usually results from an accident at a building site or a car crash and possible injuries include fractures and internal/external haemorrhage.

Following a crush injury, a number of serious complications can occur, including:
- **impaired circulation:** particularly below the injury site
- **release of toxic waste:** can affect the kidneys and lungs. If released suddenly into the circulation, they can lead to renal failure. This 'crush syndrome' can be fatal
- **shock:** once the pressure is released, tissue fluid can leak into the injured area which can rapidly lead to shock.

Treatment

Crush injury <15 minutes: quickly release casualty, monitor his vital signs, control external bleeding, immobilise any fractures, treat for shock and ensure that the emergency services have been alerted.

Crush injury >15 minutes: do not release casualty, monitor his vital signs and ensure that the emergency services have been alerted (St John Ambulance, 2002; British Red Cross, 2003).

Amputated limb or digit

Amputation can be defined as the complete or partial severing of a limb or digit (finger or toe). Causes include occupational injuries, e.g. industrial machinery and power tools, and road traffic accidents. If the amputated part is kept at 4°C, it may be possible to re-attach the amputated part within 12–24 hours.

Treatment

- If available, put on disposable gloves
- Control bleeding: apply sterile dressing and direct pressure and raise the injured part
- Monitor the casualty's vital signs
- Treat for shock if required
- Ensure the emergency services are alerted (arrange transport to hospital if it is only a digit that has been amputated and the casualty is not in shock)
- Ensure adequate care of amputated limb of digit (see below)
- Ensure that the casualty does not have anything to eat or drink (a general anaesthetic may be required in hospital)

Care of the amputated limb or digit

When caring for the injured part:
- do not wash it
- wrap in kitchen film or place in a plastic bag; then wrap in soft fabric and place on ice (ensure it does not come into contact with the ice)
- label the package: casualty's name and time of accident/injury
- hand over package to the emergency services (British Red Cross, 2003).

Do not freeze or place the amputated part in solution

Three categories of bleeding

There are three categories of bleeding: arterial, venous and capillary.

Arterial bleeding

Arterial bleeding is usually bright red in nature, due to the rich oxygenation of the red blood cells. Equally it is often of a bounding pulsation in nature. An arterial splatter or spurt is also typical, i.e. these bleeds can travel far, spraying the wall.

Venous bleeding

Venous bleeding is arguably second to arterial in the category of severity, yet more common, with the potential to lose a significant proportion of the body's circulatory volume. Venous bleeding is darker in colour than arterial bleeds, due to its deoxygenated nature. This type of bleeding usually presents as a slow trickle or is pulsatile, particularly if it is directly from source, e.g. a ruptured varicose vein.

Capillary bleeding

Capillary bleeding is minor in nature, e.g. bleeding from a graze. While bleeding may be minor and tends to be mixed with serous fluid, it is often from a wide area. Control is nevertheless simple. Infection may be the overriding consideration as a complication of this type of bleed, rather than the bleed itself.

General principles for the first aid treatment of severe bleeding

The general principles for the first aid treatment of severe bleeding are to:

- remove clothing to expose the wound
- put on disposable gloves if available
- apply direct pressure to the wound using a sterile dressing if possible or a clean pad; it may be necessary to place further pads

- if it is not possible to apply direct pressure to the wound, squeeze the edges of the wound together
- elevate the wound; raise the injured part of the body above the level of the heart to slow down blood flow to the wound (Fig. 13.5)
- ask the casualty to lie down, with the legs raised if you think that shock may develop
- ensure the emergency services are alerted
- monitor the casualty's vital signs: observe for signs of shock
- keep the casualty warm
  (Resuscitation Council UK & British Heart Foundation, 2003).

Direct pressure in the form of compressing the wound site will aid clot formation and thus stem the flow of bleeding. Dressing upon dressing should be placed over the wound until the haemorrhaging stops seeping through the dressing in question. Fresh dressings may need to be applied. The casualty or a bystander could help where appropriate.

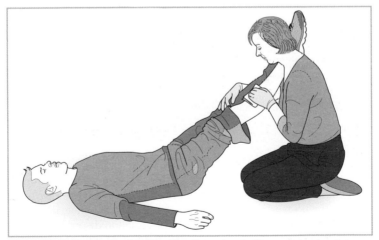

Figure 13.5 Treatment of severe bleeding: elevate the wound; raise the injured part of the body above the level of the heart to slow down blood flow to the wound

Elevating the limb above the level of the heart is also helpful. Here, gravity will help stem the flow of blood. If this involves the leg, then both legs should be raised. This is easier to manage, and will also assist with the effects of shock.

If haemorrhage is significant and control is difficult, pressure points at the femoral and brachial arteries may be compressed. This is known as indirect pressure, i.e. pressure applied away from the source of bleeding. Indirect pressure should be used in conjunction with direct pressure/compression and elevation.

Tourniquets

The use of tourniquets is controversial. Arterial tourniquets cause ischaemic injury following 90 minutes of compression. Complications include bleeding, soft tissue injury, vascular and nerve injury, and paralysis.

Tourniquets applied in the first aid setting often cause venous rather than arterial occlusion and often increase rather than decrease haemorrhage. It is therefore recommended that a tourniquet is only used as a last resort for massive haemorrhage which is not controlled by other methods and only by a person skilled in its use.

Treatment for specific bleeding

Epistaxis

Epistaxis (nose bleed) is usually caused by ruptured blood vessels on the nasal septum, close to Little's area. It is often due either to a blow to the nose or minor trauma, e.g. nose picking, sneezing. It can also complicate hypertension and coagulation disorders; in the case of the latter it can be severe and is associated with significant mortality. In the elderly, bleeding can be profuse, leading to hypovolaemic shock.

Wounds and bleeding
Treatment for specific bleeding
199

First aid treatment

- Sit the casualty down, ideally on the floor
- Ask the casualty to sit up and bend forwards at the waist; this will allow the blood to drain from the nostrils; a bowl in front of the casualty allowing blood to drip into it would be helpful
- Ask the casualty to pinch the nasal alae with the thumb and index finger (Fig. 13.6)
- Encourage the casualty to breathe through the mouth and not the nose
- Discourage swallowing because this may dislodge the accumulating clot; placing a cork between the casualty's front teeth (Trotter's method) can help to prevent swallowing
- Also ask the casualty not to speak, cough or spit, again because this may dislodge the accumulating clot
- After 10 minutes, ask the casualty to release the pressure and re-assess; if the bleeding has not stopped, reapply the pressure for another 10 minutes; repeat for a third time if necessary
- If the bleeding stops, encourage the casualty to rest; assess the vital signs; advice should be given not to pick or blow the nose and to avoid hot drinks and spicy foods for at least 24 hours
- Continued bleeding may require medical attention; if the nose bleed is severe or lasts longer than 30 minutes, take or send the casualty to hospital

Bleeding from the scalp

The scalp is inherently very vascular. Even a mild wound can result in profuse haemorrhaging, making it look far worse than it actually is.

First aid treatment

- Lay the casualty down, with the head and shoulders slightly raised
- Apply direct pressure using a pad; secure the dressing with a roller bandage
- Monitor the casualty's vital signs; in particular conscious level (AVPU, see p. 24)
- Take or send the casualty to hospital

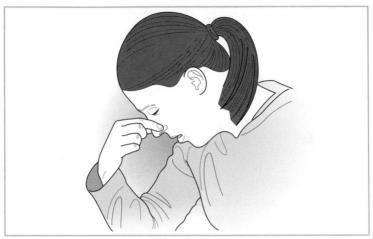

Figure 13.6 Epistaxis: ask the casualty to pinch the nasal alae with the thumb and index figure. Reproduced with permission from O'Shea, Principles of Practice of Trauma Nursing, Elsevier Ltd

Bleeding from the mouth

Bleeding from the mouth can be profuse and look alarming. Causes include a tooth extraction and cuts to the lips and gums. The casualty may feel as if he is choking on his own blood or saliva, and airway compromise is a potential complication. It can be difficult to treat, due to poor access, poor lighting and a moist environment.

First aid treatment

- Sit the casualty down
- Ask the casualty to tilt the head slightly towards the injured side, thus enabling blood to drain out of the mouth

- Place a sterile pad over the wound and ask the casualty to apply pressure for 10 minutes, then re-assess
- If the bleeding is from a tooth socket, place a gauze pad that is sufficiently thick to prevent the casualty's teeth from touching over the socket and ask the casualty to bite down
- Advise the casualty not to rinse the mouth out (may dislodge clot) and to avoid hot drinks for 12 hours
- Seek medical or dental help (as appropriate) if the bleeding has not stopped after 30 minutes

Bleeding from the abdomen

Abdominal injuries are associated with high mortality and morbidity because the potential for serious complications is often underestimated, consequently significant injuries are overlooked and remain undetected.

Causes of abdominal injuries include road traffic accidents, crush accidents, knife wounds and shootings. Abdominal trauma can be difficult to diagnose or determine the extent of injury. There is also a significant risk of infection from peritonitis, the puncturing instrument or from a protruding bowel.

First aid treatment

- Help the casualty to lie down
- Place dressing (sterile if possible) over the wound
- Alert the emergency services
- Monitor the casualty's vital signs; observe for signs of shock
- If the casualty starts to cough or vomit, apply pressure to the dressing to prevent the bowel pushing through the wound and becoming exposed
- If the bowel is protruding: cover with kitchen film or a plastic bag to alleviate the risk of drying the bowel and to reduce infection

Conclusion

There are many different types of wounds. This chapter has discussed the treatment of different wounds and embedded objects. It is important to recognise which wounds can be managed at home and which will require medical attention. The treatment of bleeding has also been described. A key priority is ensuring that the risk of infection is minimised, both to the rescuer and the casualty. If possible, sterile gloves should be worn.

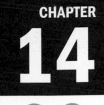

Burns and scalds

Introduction

Each year there are approximately 250 000 burn injuries in the UK (Hudspith & Rayatt, 2004) and 1.25 million in the USA (Sheridan, 2003). Annually, there are approximately 300 burn-related deaths in the UK (Hettiaratchy & Dwiewulski, 2004a) and 3700 in the USA (National Safety Council, 1999).

High-risk groups include infants and young children, elderly persons and young persons in industrial occupations. A large number of burns occur at home, work and recreational areas. The key causes of household burns are kettles/steam, hot oil or fat, and hot drinks.

The aim of this chapter is to understand the first aid treatment of burns and scalds.

Chapter objectives
At the end of the chapter the reader will be able to:

- **Outline the structure and functions of the skin**

- **Discuss the causes and types of burns**

- **Describe the classification and characteristics of burns**

- **Outline the first aid treatment of burns**

- **Discuss the treatment of chemical burns and electrical burns**

- **Identify when medical attention for burns is required**

Structure and functions of the skin

Structure
• •

The skin, the largest organ in the body, consists of two main layers: the epidermis (outer layer) and dermis. The nerve endings responsible for the sensation of touch and temperature are located in the dermis. Structures within the skin include sweat glands, hair follicles and sebaceous glands and there is a layer of subcutaneous fat between the skin and underlying structures.

Functions
• •

Functions of the skin include:
• thermoregulation
• protection against infection
• protection against ultraviolet rays
• waterproofing
• sensation of touch
• absorption and excretion
• synthesis of vitamin D
  (Taylor, 2001).

The skin acts as a barrier to the environment; without it there is a risk of infection, hypothermia and body fluid can be lost. Burns that affect >15% of total body surface area in adults, or >10% in children or elderly persons over 70 years of age, can lead to shock: IV fluid resuscitation and intensive burn care will be required.

Causes and types of burns

Types and possible causes
• •

Table 14.1 details the different types of burns, including the possible causes.

Table 14.1 Types of burns and their causes

Burn type	Possible causes
Dry burn	Flames, contact with hot objects or friction
Scald Hot cooking oil	Hot fluid, steam or hot fat
Electrical burn	Low and high voltage currents, lightning strike
Cold injury	Frostbite, contact with freezing product
Chemical burn	Domestic chemicals, e.g. bleach and industrial chemicals including fumes/corrosive gases
Radiation burn	Usually sunburn or over-exposure to sunlamp ultraviolet rays (Butcher, 2001)

Sources: Bosworth, 1997; St John Ambulance, St Andrew's Ambulance, British Red Cross, 2000

Incidence and causes of burns by age

- **Infants/small children (<4 years) 20%:** 70% caused by scalds due to the spilling of hot fluids or hot bathing water; flame injuries are now less common due to the changes in the design and material of nightwear

- **Children/adolescents (5–14 years) 10%:** in teenagers electrocution and involvement with unlawful activities involving accelerants, e.g. petrol are the most common causes

- **Working age adults (15–64 years) 60%:** mainly due to flame injuries; approximately 30% are work related

- **Elderly adults (65 years and over) 10%:** reduced mobility, decreased dexterity and slowed reactions can render elderly adults susceptible to scalds, contact and flame burns (Hettiaratchy & Dwiewulski, 2004a)

Classification and characteristics of burns

Burns can be classified into two groups depending upon burn depth: partial thickness burns (superficial, superficial dermal and deep dermal) and full thickness burns. The terms first, second and third degree burns are rarely used now because they are deemed too subjective and are open to misinterpretation.

Burn depth is related to the amount of energy delivered in the injury and to the relative thickness of the skin (the dermis is thinner in children and the elderly). Table 14.2 details the different classifications of burns and skin structures involved, together with the key characteristics.

Estimating the extent of the burn injury

Estimating the extent of the burn injury is the first step in estimating the burn injury severity. There are three commonly used methods for assessing the burn area:

1. **Palmar surface:** the casualty's palm (including fingers) is approximately 0.8% of the total body surface area; palmar surface can be used for small burns (<15% of total surface area) and very large burns (>85% of total surface area) (Hettiaratchy & Papini, 2004).
2. **Wallace rule of nines:** quick and easy way of estimating medium to large burns in adults – the body is divided into areas divisible by 9 (Kyle & Wallace, 1951); it is inaccurate in children <14 years.
3. **Lund & Bowder chart:** provides a formula that can be used in children (Lund & Bowder, 1944).

Simple erythema (reddening of the skin) should not be included when estimating burn area

First aid treatment of burns

The aims of first aid are to stop the burning process, cool the burn, provide pain relief and cover the burn. Consensus guidelines that incorporate a nine-step approach to the pre-hospital management of a burns patient are available (Table 14.3). The first aid treatment of burns will now be outlined with specific reference to these guidelines.

Table 14.2 Burn depth	
Burn depth and skin structures involved	**Key characteristics**
Superficial (epidermis)	Skin: dry, intact, red, painful Blanches under pressure Minimal tissue damage Usually no blisters
Superficial dermal (epidermis and superficial dermis)	Blisters immediately (pink/red wound under blister) Red in areas, moist and exuding Brisk capillary refill Blanches under pressure Painful Sensitive to changes in temperature
Deep dermal (Epidermis and deep dermis)	Pale, white, large easily liftable blisters may be present Initially less moist Capillary refill difficult to assess Slightly painful with areas that are insensate – sensitive to deep pressure but not a pin prick
Full thickness (epidermis and dermis, subcutaneous tissue; deeper structures may be affected if chemical or electrical burn)	Waxy white, deep red, grey or leathery Minimal or no pain in wound – no response to pressure or temperature Wound may have less deep and painful peripheries

Sources: Fowler, 2003; Hettiaratchy & Papini, 2004

SAFE approach

The SAFE acronym can be used to remind the rescuer as to the initial priorities in the care of the casualty:
- Shout or call for help
- Assess the scene for dangers to either the rescuer or the patient

Burns and scalds
First aid treatment of burns
209

> **Table 14.3** Consensus guidelines on the pre-hospital approach to burns patient management (Allison & Porter, 2004)
>
> SAFE approach
> Stop the burning process
> Cooling
> Covering/dressing
> Assessment of AcBC
> Assessment of burns severity
> Cannulation (and fluids)
> Analgesia
> Transport

- <u>F</u>ree from danger
- <u>E</u>valuate the patient.

Stop the burning process

Remove the heat source. Remove burnt clothing (unless it is stuck to the casualty) as soon as possible because it can retain heat. Adherent material, e.g. nylon, should be left on. Remove any jewellery, which may become constrictive.

If the casualty's clothing is on fire, have the casualty 'stop, drop and roll' and soak the flames with water or smother them with a blanket. Roll the casualty over and over to put the flames out.

Cooling

Cooling the burn wound is effective if it is undertaken within 20 minutes of the injury. By removing heat and preventing burn progression, cooling a burn has many beneficial effects:
- halts the burning process
- reduces pain

- reduces oedema
- cleanses the wound and reduces infection rates
- reduces the depth of injury
- reduces the need for grafting
- speeds up the healing process.

Cool running tap water is adequate for cooling. Iced water should not be used because the resultant vasoconstriction could cause burn progression and additional local injury due to ischaemia. Excessive cooling with iced water and the use of ice packs could cause profound hypothermia, particularly in children. As well as cooling the wound, attempts should be made to keep the patient warm.

Cool the burn wound but warm the patient

Covering/dressing

Cover the burn wound to prevent infection. Minimising the risk of infection will promote wound healing. Polyvinyl chloride film (Cling film) is ideal in the first aid setting for dressing a burn wound as it is:

- basically sterile (as long as the first few centimetres are discarded)
- pliable
- non-adherent
- impermeable – acts as a barrier
- transparent for wound inspection (Hudspith & Rayatt, 2004).

If using Cling film, it is important to lay it on the burn rather than wrapping it around it; this is particularly important on limbs because subsequent swelling may lead to constriction. If Cling film is not available, a clean cotton sheet could be used. Hand burns can be covered by a clear plastic bag.

Refrain from using topical creams at this stage because they may interfere with subsequent assessment of the burn. Paramedics will often use a cooling gel, e.g. Burnshield, to cool the burn and relieve the pain.

Blisters should be left intact – lancing a blister in less than sterile conditions increases the risk of infection. In addition, leaving blisters intact may also be beneficial to the patient.

Assessment of AcBC

It is important to remember that the casualty may have other injuries coexistent with the burn injury. The assessment of airway with cervical spine stabilisation, breathing and circulation may also be pertinent.

Assessment of burn severity

A quick assessment of the burn severity is helpful (see above). Other important features of the burn to define include:
- time of burn injury
- mechanism of injury – flame, clothes or patient caught fire, flash burn, scald, electrical, chemical
- burn within a confined space – possible inhalation injury
- possible non-accidental injury in children and elderly persons.

If possible maintain accurate records (Ashworth et al, 2001).

For all burns and scalds on young children: seek medical attention
In all cases if the burn or scald is severe: seek medical attention

Cannulation (and fluids)

Cannulation and IV fluid resuscitation may be started by the emergency services.

Analgesia

In the first aid setting, pain relief is best accomplished by cooling and covering the burned area (see above).

Burns and scalds
212
First aid treatment of burns

Transport

All treatment should be undertaken with the aim of reducing on-scene times and delivering the patient to the appropriate treatment centre, e.g. the nearest appropriate Accident and Emergency department.

Thermal inhalation injury

Thermal inhalation injury remains a major source of morbidity and mortality secondary to early airway obstruction and bronchospasm. In particular, it can be associated with a burn injury within a confined space. Clinical features of smoke inhalation and thermal injury to the respiratory tract include:
- altered level of consciousness
- facial burn
- burns to the oropharynx
- stridor
- hoarseness
- soot evident in the nostrils or sputum
- expiratory rhonchi
- dysphagia
- dribbling, drooling of saliva
  (Robertson & Fenton, 2000).

If inhalation injury is suspected, dial 999 for an ambulance and inform the control officer that inhalation injury is suspected. The patient may require urgent advanced airway intervention, e.g. intubation

While waiting for the ambulance:
- take steps to improve the casualty's air supply, e.g. loosen clothing around the neck
- offer ice or small sips of cold water to help reduce swelling and/or pain
- monitor ABC.

Burns and scalds
Electrical and chemical burns
213

Paediatric burns

Along with the elderly, children suffer the highest morbidity and mortality rates from burn injuries.

The effect of a burn injury on a child and the parents/family cannot be underestimated; parents can find themselves in utter turmoil after a traumatic, often preventable, incident.

The possibility of non-accidental injury should always be considered. Approximately 3–10% of paediatric burns are due to non-accidental injury, and it is more common in young children (<3 years) (Hettiaratchy & Dziewulski, 2004b).

Electrical and chemical burns

Electrical burns

Electrical burns account for approximately 3–4% of burns unit admissions. The severity of electrical injuries can vary widely from an unpleasant tingling sensation to thermal burns and even cardiopulmonary arrest.

Burns can result from both low and high voltage injuries. Although high voltage injuries are the most dangerous, nevertheless, fatal electrocutions can be caused by low-voltage household current. It would be helpful to distinguish between flash electrical burns and contact electrical burns.

- Flash electrical burns: produce superficial charring of the skin; usually less severe than it looks and heals well unless there has been an associated burn injury due to clothing that has caught fire
- Contact electrical burns: result from an electrical current passing through bodily tissues and damaging tissue in its passage; these burns are worse than they look; 'entry' and 'exit' points are created and a particular concern after an electrical injury is the need for cardiac monitoring.

First aid treatment of electrical burns:
- ensure it is safe to approach
- apply cold water to sites of injury
- apply dressings (see above)
- monitor ABC while waiting for the emergency services
  (St John Ambulance, St Andrew's Ambulance, British Red Cross, 2002).

Chemical burns

Chemical burns are usually caused by industrial accidents, but may also occur with household chemical products. Chemical burns can cause continuing tissue destruction and systemic toxicity.

Early treatment with copious lavage is paramount. Prolonged irrigation may be required.

First aid treatment of chemical burns while awaiting the emergency services:
- ensure it is safe to approach – put on gloves if available, ventilate the area to disperse fumes and if possible seal the chemical container; it may be necessary to move the casualty (St John Ambulance, St Andrew's Ambulance, British Red Cross, 2002)
- gently remove any contaminated clothing
- apply large amounts of cold water to burn site
- apply dressings (see above)
- monitor ABC while waiting for the emergency services
- if possible, find out the name of the chemical and inform the emergency services.

Burns requiring medical attention

Medical attention should be sought for all serious burns including:
- full-thickness burns
- burns involving the face, hands, feet or genitalia

- burns that extend around an arm or leg
- partial thickness burns >1% of the body surface (approximately the area of the casualty's palm)
- all superficial burns >5% of the body surface (approximately the area of the casualty's palm × 5)
- burns with a mixed pattern of varying depths
  (St John Ambulance, St Andrew's Ambulance, British Red Cross, 2002).

Conclusion

Each year there are approximately 250 000 burn injuries and 300 burns-related deaths in the UK. High-risk groups include infants and young children, elderly persons and young persons in industrial occupations. Most burns occur at home, work and recreational areas. This chapter has provided an overview of the first aid treatment of burns.

Musculoskeletal injuries

Co-written with Mark Gillett

Musculoskeletal injuries

Introduction

Injuries to the bones and soft tissues of the locomotor system can cause significant morbidity and mortality, ranging from the pain and inconvenience of a lateral ligament injury of the ankle, to the potentially life-threatening sequelae of a fractured pelvis.

The aim of this chapter is to understand the first aid treatment of musculoskeletal injuries.

Chapter objectives
At the end of the chapter the reader will be able to:

- **List the common terms used in musculoskeletal injuries**

- **Describe the examination of a casualty with a musculoskeletal injury**

- **Discuss the classification of fractures**

- **Describe the common signs and symptoms of a fracture**

- **Describe the general care of a casualty with a fracture**

- **Discuss the treatment for specific fractures and dislocations**

- **Discuss the management of a suspected spinal injury**

- **Outline the treatment for a sprained ankle**

Common terms in musculoskeletal injury

Common terms in musculoskeletal injury:
- Fracture: a disruption of the cortex of a living bone
- Dislocation: the components of a joint are completely separated without an accompanying fracture
- Subluxation: the components of a joint are incompletely separated without an accompanying fracture
- Sprain: a tear of a ligament
- Tendonitis: inflammation of a tendon.

Examination of a casualty with a musculoskeletal injury

After ensuring it is safe to approach, undertake the ABCDE assessment, regardless of any apparent musculoskeletal injury. It is easy to become distracted by an obvious fractured femur and overlook a concomitant injury that will lead to an earlier threat to life, e.g. upper airway compromise.

Then examine the musculoskeletal injury:
- look for obvious deformity, swelling, bleeding or protruding bone
- feel for crepitus, swelling or abnormal movement
- move (actively and passively) the affected joints: initially ask the casualty to move the joint (active movement), then assess the range and quality of movement, if this is felt appropriate (passive movement).

Classification of fractures

A fracture is defined as a disruption of the cortex of a living bone. The following subtypes are frequently referred to in clinical practice.

- Simple fracture: bone is broken into two pieces (Fig. 15.1); the fracture can be further described as transverse, spiral or oblique according to its shape.

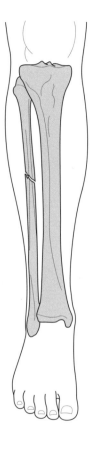

Figure 15.1 Simple fracture: bone is broken into two pieces. Reproduced with permission from O'Shea, Principles & Practice of Trauma Nursing, Elsevier Ltd

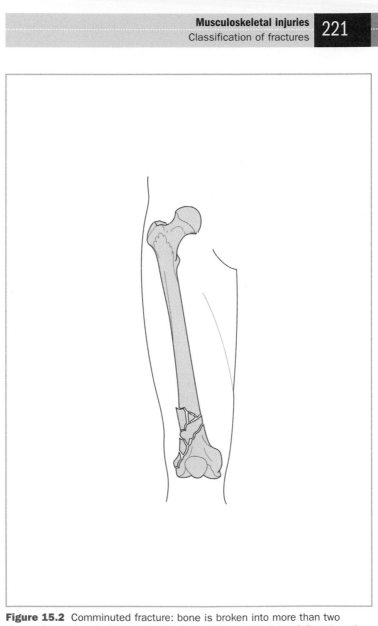

Figure 15.2 Comminuted fracture: bone is broken into more than two pieces. Reproduced with permission from O'Shea, Principles & Practice of Trauma Nursing, Elsevier Ltd

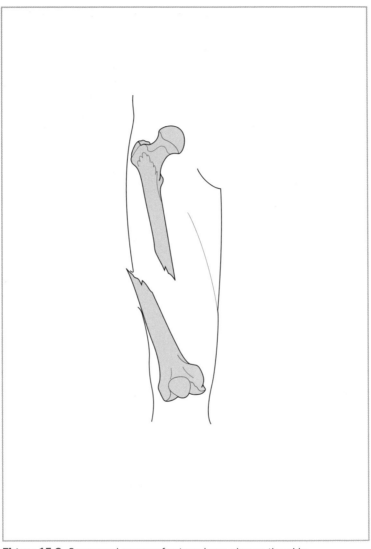

Figure 15.3 Compound or open fracture: bone pierces the skin.
Reproduced with permission from O'Shea, Principles & Practice of Trauma
Nursing, Elsevier Ltd

- Comminuted fracture: the bone is broken into more than two pieces (Fig. 15.2).
- Closed fracture: bone does not pierce the skin.
- Compound or open fracture: bone pierces the skin (Fig. 15.3).
- Greenstick fracture: occurs in children when the bone bends, causing one aspect of the cortex to break while the other remains intact.
- Pathological fracture: bone is weakened by another pathology, most commonly metastases or osteoporosis, and is prone to pathological fractures. If the tensile strength of the bone is grossly reduced, the bone may fracture with a minimal amount of trauma.
- Stress fractures occur secondary to overuse, either acutely or over a longer period of time, predominantly in the lower limb.

Common signs and symptoms of a fracture

Common signs and symptoms of a fracture include:
- history of impact or trauma
- swelling, bruising or deformity
- pain on movement
- numbness or tingling
- visible wound or injury
- crepitus (grating of bones)
- circulatory shock if the femur or pelvis is affected.

General care of a casualty with a fracture

The general care of a casualty with a fracture involves supporting the injured limb, arranging transfer to hospital, monitoring the casualty and treating shock.

Supporting the injured limb

- Unless it is unsafe to do so, leave the casualty in the position found
- If a cervical spinal injury is suspected, support the head and neck at all times to prevent further injury
- Ask the casualty to remain still; movement of a fracture can be very painful, can increase damage to surrounding tissues and may precipitate shock
- Secure and support the injured limb
- Cover any wound with a sterile wound dressing (preferable) or a clean, non-fluffy pad; if bleeding is present, apply pressure

Arranging transfer to hospital

- The site and the extent of the injury will determine how the casualty should be transferred to hospital, e.g. in the case of an arm injury, a car journey may be possible
- If an injury to the spine or neck is suspected, always alert the emergency services

Monitoring the casualty

- Monitor the casualty's vital signs
- Frequently check for the presence or absence of distal pulses and sensation; pulses that are impalpable should be compared to the contralateral side in order to judge if a pre-existing pathology may be complicating the situation
- Check capillary refill distal to the fracture and compare with the contralateral side

Treating shock

- Treat for shock and if necessary raise the legs

Do not raise the injured limb if this causes the casualty more pain

Treatment of an open fracture

Open fractures are at high risk of infection and can be associated with gross soft tissue damage, severe haemorrhage or vascular injury. The vast majority of open fractures occur on the limbs and the resulting degree of soft tissue injury correlates well with subsequent infection rates.

Cover the wound with a sterile wound dressing (preferable) or a clean, non-fluffy pad and immobilise the fracture. If bleeding is present, apply pressure.

Treatment of a closed fracture

Effective immobilisation of the fracture site is the key to achieving adequate analgesia. This is achieved most simply in the lower limb by binding it to the contralateral side. Box splints also provide simple and effective immobilisation for lower limb injuries, while broad arm and high arm slings have their place in the treatment of upper limb injuries.

Treatment for specific fractures and dislocations

Fractured clavicle

A fractured clavicle is usually caused by either a direct injury or from falling onto the outstretched hand or point of the shoulder. It is commonly associated with sporting activities and often in young people. A significant deceleration injury could also be the cause of a fractured clavicle (and bruising of the chest wall) due to the wearing of a seat-belt.

There will probably be pain, swelling and deformity of the shoulder and the casualty often presents supporting the arm (usually the elbow) on the injured side and inclining the head towards the injured side (to help relax muscles and relieve pain).

First aid treatment:

- help the casualty to sit down

- lay the arm of the injured side diagonally across the chest, so that the fingertips touch the opposite shoulder and ask the casualty to support the elbow on the affected side with the other hand

- apply an elevation sling to support the arm on the affected side; some soft padding between the arm and body will make the casualty feel more comfortable

- apply a broad-fold bandage (Fig. 15.4) to strap the arm to the chest, tying the knot on the uninjured side

- arrange to transfer the casualty to hospital in the sitting position (St John Ambulance, 2002; British Red Cross, 2003).

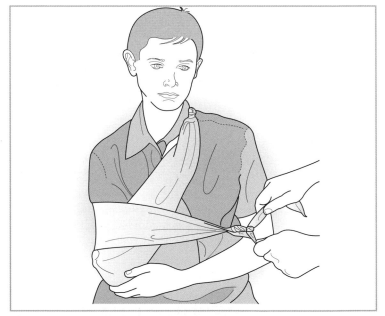

Figure 15.4 Application of a broad fold bandage

Dislocation of the shoulder

Dislocation of the shoulder is common. Anatomically, the shoulder is a ball and socket synovial joint that relies heavily on the joint capsule and the surrounding rotator cuff muscles for stability. The fact that the shoulder has exceptional mobility accounts for it being the most commonly dislocated large joint in the body. Three major types of shoulder dislocation are recognised:

- anterior dislocation
- posterior dislocation
- luxatio erecta (true inferior dislocation).

Anterior dislocations are by far the most common type and generally occur after a fall or trauma to the upper limb with the shoulder abducted and externally rotated. Clinically, an anterior dislocation gives the shoulder a squared-off appearance, enabling a clinical diagnosis to be made. The casualty will complain of pain and will be unwilling to move the shoulder.

Assessment of sensation over the deltoid muscle is essential to evaluate whether the axillary nerve, which runs around the surgical neck of the humerus, has been damaged. The presence of distal pulses and capillary refill in the hand should also be assessed. First aid treatment essentially involves immobilisation.

First aid treatment:
- help the casualty to sit down
- lay the arm of the injured side across the body in a position that is most comfortable for the casualty
- ask the casualty to support the hand of the injured side
- apply a triangular arm sling to support the arm on the affected side; some soft padding between the arm and body will make the casualty feel more comfortable
- apply a broad-fold bandage (see Fig. 15.4) to strap the arm to the chest, tying the knot on the uninjured side
- arrange to transfer the casualty to hospital in the sitting position (St John Ambulance, 2002; British Red Cross, 2003).

Flail chest

A flail chest is where two or more ribs are fractured in two or more places so that they are not attached to the rib cage and do not move in conjunction with it during inspiration and expiration. This portion of the chest wall is called 'flail' and appears to be free-floating.

Paradoxical breathing can occur, whereby the flail segment moves in an opposite direction to the rest of the rib cage during each respiratory phase. On inspiration a flail segment moves inwards, and on expiration, outwards. This can lead to a reduced tidal volume and compromised breathing. A flail chest will cause hypoxia.

First aid treatment:
* reassure the casualty and monitor vital signs
* leaning the casualty towards the injured side will help with breathing, thus facilitating unobstructed movement of the uninjured lung
* alert the emergency services.

Fractured humerus

A fractured humerus usually results from a fall onto an outstretched hand or onto the elbow. Its occurrence is much more common in the elderly.

First aid treatment:
* help the casualty to sit down
* lay the forearm of the injured side horizontally across the chest, in the position that is most comfortable for the casualty
* ask the casualty to support the elbow
* apply a triangular arm sling to support the arm on the affected side; some soft padding between the arm and body will make the casualty feel more comfortable
* apply a broad-fold bandage (see Fig. 15.4) to strap the arm to the chest, tying the knot on the uninjured side

• arrange to transfer the casualty to hospital in the sitting position
(St John Ambulance, 2002; British Red Cross, 2003).

Dislocated elbow

When the elbow is dislocated, there will be a disruption in the
normal triangular anatomical relationship between the epicondyles
and the olecranon. If it is possible to bend the elbow, the first aid
treatment is as follows:
• help the casualty to sit down
• lay the forearm of the injured side horizontally across the chest, in a
position that is most comfortable for the casualty
• ask the casualty to support the elbow
• check (and regularly monitor) the pulse in the wrist of the injured side: if
the pulse is not present, gently straighten the elbow until it returns and
then maintain and support this position
• apply a triangular arm sling to support the arm and elbow on the
affected side; some soft padding between the arm and body will make
the casualty feel more comfortable
• apply a broad-fold bandage (see Fig. 15.4) to strap the arm to the chest,
tying the knot on the uninjured side
• arrange to transfer the casualty to hospital in the sitting position
(St John Ambulance, 2002; British Red Cross, 2003).

If it is not possible to bend the elbow:
• help the casualty to lie down
• immobilise the injured arm using such supports as cushions or rolled up
towels
• alert the emergency services
• check for (and regularly monitor) the radial pulse.

Fractured radius, ulna or wrist

A fractured radius, ulna or wrist usually results from a fall onto an
outstretched hand or onto the elbow.

The common Colles' fracture is a fracture of the radius within 2.5 cm of the wrist joint with posterior displacement and posterior angulation of the distal fragment. It is particularly common from middle age onwards with the classical dinner-fork deformity after falling on an outstretched hand. The increased frequency in post-menopausal women is caused by osteoporosis.

First aid treatment:
- help the casualty to sit down
- gently lay the forearm across the chest, in a position that is most comfortable for the casualty
- ask the casualty to support the forearm
- apply a triangular arm sling to support the arm on the affected side; some soft padding, e.g. a folded towel, between the arm and body will make the casualty feel more comfortable
- apply a broad-fold bandage (see Fig. 15.4) to strap the arm to the chest, tying the knot on the uninjured side
- arrange to transfer the casualty to hospital in the sitting position (St John Ambulance, 2002; British Red Cross, 2003).

Fractures in the hand, carpals and metacarpals

Fractures in the hand, carpals and metacarpals are often caused by crush injuries. The fractures may be open with severe bleeding and swelling. It is often helpful to compare the injured hand with the uninjured hand, because sometimes deformities may not be very obvious.

First aid treatment:
- help the casualty to sit down
- if possible, remove any rings from the affected hand/fingers
- raise the casualty's hand and support the arm in an elevation sling
- apply a broad-fold bandage to strap the arm to the chest, tying the knot on the uninjured side
- arrange to transfer the casualty to hospital in the sitting position (St John Ambulance, 2002; British Red Cross, 2003).

Fracture of the pelvis

Fractures of the pelvis are relatively common and in road traffic accidents are often associated with multiple injuries. Associated damage to the urinary tract is common. They are potentially fatal due to haemorrhage into the peritoneal and retro-peritoneal cavities. Major pelvic fractures often occur after high velocity trauma when the treatment priorities depend on the primary survey findings.

The casualty will not be able to walk or even stand and will have pain in the pelvic region; in addition, he may want to pass urine (frank haematuria may be evident).

First aid treatment:
* help the casualty to lie down supine
* if possible keep the legs straight; however, it may be more comfortable to bend the knees slightly and place some padding such as a cushion or rolled up clothing to support them
* alert the emergency services
* immobilise the legs (Fig. 15.5): place some padding between the ankles and knees and then tie the ankles and feet, then the knees together
* monitor the casualty's vital signs, particularly for signs of shock (St John Ambulance, 2002)

Fractures of the hip and femur

Hip fractures usually occur in the elderly with decreased bone density. The classical presentation is of a shortened, externally rotated lower limb, although undisplaced fractures may not lead to this deformity in the leg.

Fracture of the femur can result following high velocity trauma or after comparatively trivial injuries in a casualty with osteopenic bone. The injured leg may look shorter than the uninjured one and there may be some rotation.

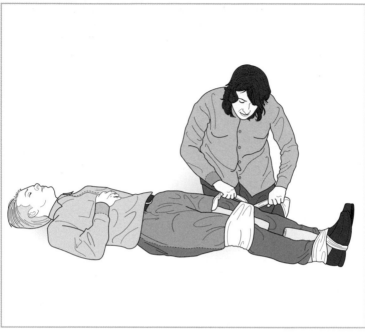

Figure 15.5 Immobilisation of the legs: place some padding between the ankles and then tie the ankles and feet, and then the knees

Following a femoral fracture, approximately 1500 ml of blood can be lost and the casualty is at risk of hypovolaemic shock. In open fractures, the blood loss could be considerably more.

First aid treatment:
- help the casualty to lie down supine
- gently straighten the lower leg; it may be necessary to apply traction at the ankle. Keep the leg still
- alert the emergency services
- if there is an open wound, apply a dressing (sterile if possible)

- if the arrival of the emergency services is going to be delayed, immobilise the legs (see Fig. 15.5): place some padding between the ankles and knees and then tie the ankles and feet, then the knees together
- monitor the casualty's vital signs, particularly for signs of shock.

Fractures of the tibia/fibula

Fractures of the tibia/fibula are common, particularly in footballers and motorcyclists. There will be localised pain, swelling, bruising and deformity of the injured leg. There may be an open wound, particularly if the tibia is injured.

First aid treatment:
- help the casualty to lie down supine
- alert the emergency services
- if there is an open wound, cover it with a sterile wound dressing (preferable) or a clean, non-fluffy pad; if bleeding is present, apply pressure
- support the injured leg by placing one hand above and the other below the break (Fig. 15.6)
- if the arrival of the emergency services is going to be delayed, immobilise the injured limb by placing some padding between the two ankles and two knees and then tying the ankle, feet and knees together
- monitor the casualty's vital signs.

Fractures of the ankle

Fractures of the ankle are common, usually following an inversion injury to the ankle, where the sole of the foot rotates medially and the lateral structures of the ankle are stretched while the medial structures are compressed. The casualty will complain of pain in the injured foot, and there will be swelling.

First aid treatment:
- help the casualty to lie down supine

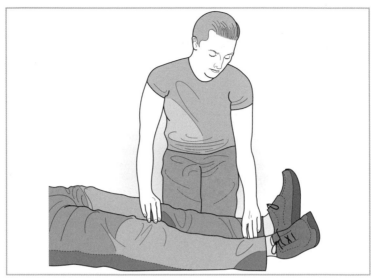

Figure 15.6 Immobilisation of the tibia/fibula: support the injured leg by placing one hand above and the other below the break

- support the injured leg by placing one hand above and the other below the break
- arrange transfer to hospital
- monitor the casualty's vital signs.

Fractures of the foot, tarsals and metatarsals

Fractures of the foot and metatarsals are usually caused by a crushing injury. It is important to be aware that multiple metatarsal or tarsal fractures can precipitate gross foot oedema, which may produce an acute compartment syndrome. The casualty will have difficulty walking and will find it painful to weight-bear on the injured foot.

First aid treatment:
- help the casualty to lie or sit down
- elevate and support the affected foot, to reduce swelling
- apply a cold compress or ice pack to reduce swelling and relieve pain
- arrange transfer to hospital.

Suspected spinal injury

If a spinal injury is suspected, particular care must be taken to maintain the head, neck and chest in the neutral position. Failure to protect the cervical spine may result in tetraplegia.

The mechanism of the injury will lead to suspicion of a spinal injury, e.g.
- road traffic accident
- diving into the shallow end of a pool and hitting the bottom
- falling from a height, e.g. off a ladder
- head injury
- horse-riding accident
- in a collapsed rugby scrum.

The casualty may complain of back pain or tenderness. If there is injury to the spinal cord, the casualty may complain of loss of sensation, burning or tingling in the extremities. Urinary and faecal incontinence and respiratory difficulties may also be evident. The spinal cord is usually damaged in the cervical region.

Treatment

If the casualty is conscious:
- leave the casualty in the position found
- maintain the head, neck and chest in the neutral position (Fig. 15.7A); this will improve the airway and reduce deformity of the spine, thus helping to relieve pressure on the spinal cord and arteries

- ask a bystander to place rolled-up clothing, cushions etc, either side of the casualty's head, to provide additional support
- avoid any unnecessary movement of the head and neck
- ensure the emergency services are alerted
- monitor the casualty's vital signs.

If the casualty is unconscious:
- leave the casualty in the position found
- maintain the head, neck and chest in the neutral position (Fig. 10.4); this will improve the airway and reduce deformity of the spine, thus helping to relieve pressure on the spinal cord and arteries
- to open the airway, use the jaw thrust manoeuvre
- avoid any unnecessary movement of the head and neck
- ensure the emergency services are alerted
- monitor the casualty's vital signs
- ask a bystander to place rolled-up clothing, cushions etc, either side of the casualty's head, to provide additional support.

The airway takes priority over cervical spine protection, i.e. the casualty should not remain with a compromised airway because of the fear of possibly injuring the cervical spine

Log-rolling the casualty

If it is necessary to move the casualty into the lateral position, the log-roll technique (Fig. 15.7A & B) is recommended. The following procedure for log-rolling is based on guidelines from the American College of Surgeons (2004):
- apply gentle, inline immobilisation to the casualty's head
- gently straighten out the casualty's arms and place next to the torso, with the palms inwards
- carefully straighten the casualty's legs and place in neutral alignment with the spine

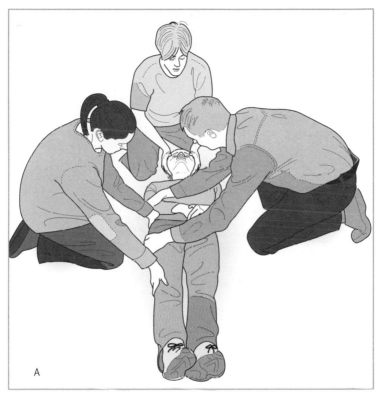

Figure 15.7A Log-roll technique 1

- ensuring everyone works together, direct the helpers to roll the casualty, ensuring that the casualty's head, torso and toes are maintained in a straight line at all times.

The above procedure assumes that cervical collars, spinal boards etc are not available, but it is essential to roll the casualty onto the side.

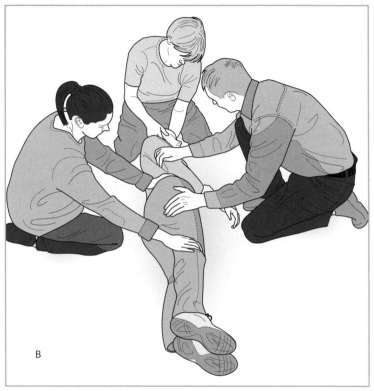

Figure 15.7B Log-roll technique 2

Four persons are required for the procedure:

- Person 1: to maintain manual, inline mobilisation of the casualty's head and neck

- Person 2: for the torso, including the pelvis and hips

- Person 3: for the pelvis and legs

- Person 4: to direct the procedure (if there are only three persons helping, the person at the head end should direct the procedure).

Sprained ankle

Soft tissue injuries (traumatic injuries to ligaments and tendons) are grossly underestimated by the general public. They can lead to prolonged periods of pain, immobility and absence from employment. The most common injury encountered is a sprained ankle.

A sprained ankle is a sprain of the lateral ligament complex of the ankle following traumatic inversion at the sub-talar joint. It can cause significant morbidity including functional instability, chronic pain, stiffness and recurrent swelling; the dominant ankle is more likely to be involved. Ankle sprain injuries account for 600 000 attendances each year at Accident & Emergency Departments in the UK.

The aim of first aid treatment in the short term is to relieve pain and reduce swelling, and in the long term is to reduce the duration of morbidity.

Treatment

The acronym RICE describes the standard first aid treatment:

Rest: short-term rest eases discomfort and does not increase morbidity

Ice: apply ice for first 24 hours intermittently: 20 minutes at a time every 4 hours. This will reduce pain and swelling

Compression: apply padding and firm bandaging to reducing swelling

Elevation: elevate the affected limb (above the waist) to reduce swelling, even while asleep (Evans & Burke, 1995).

Conclusion

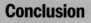

Injuries to the bones and soft tissues of the locomotor system can cause significant morbidity and mortality, ranging from the pain and inconvenience of a lateral ligament injury of the ankle, to the potentially life-threatening sequelae of a fractured pelvis. In this chapter, an overview of the first aid treatment of musculoskeletal injuries has been provided.

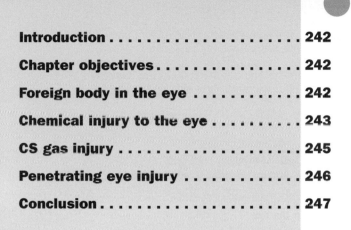

Eye injuries

Introduction

Eye injuries are, at the very least, irritating and painful for the casualty. Some can potentially be serious; even a superficial graze to the cornea can cause scarring resulting in permanent damage and deterioration in the casualty's vision. Prompt and appropriate first aid can be very beneficial.

The aim of this chapter is to understand the first aid treatment of eye injuries.

Chapter objectives
At the end of the chapter the reader will be able to discuss the treatment for a:

- **Foreign body in the eye**

- **Chemical injury to the eye**

- **CS gas injury**

- **Penetrating eye injury**

Foreign body in the eye

A foreign body in the eye, e.g. a speck of dust, grit, eyelash, can be very irritating for the casualty. The treatment depends on whether the foreign body is loose or adherent.

Treatment

- Ask the casualty to sit down, facing the light

- Stand behind the casualty and using the finger and thumb, gently separate the eyelids and examine the eye
- Ask the casualty to look left, right, up and down
- Loose foreign body: irrigate the eye with clean water (or sterile eyewash)
- Adherent foreign body: remove using a cotton wool bud or the edge of a piece of cardboard

Chemical injury to the eye

All chemical injuries to the eye can potentially cause blindness. Alkali injuries to the eyes can be particularly devastating and are much more serious than acid injuries. The speed at which the initial irrigation of the eye begins has the greatest influence on the prognosis and outcome of eye burns (Kuckelkorn et al, 2002). Prolonged irrigation will be required.

Signs and symptoms

- Painful eye
- Redness and swelling around the eye
- Inability to open the eye
- Copious watering of the eye
- History suggestive of chemical injury
  (St John Ambulance, 2002)

Treatment

The priority is to irrigate the eye so that the chemical is diluted and dispersed. The eye should be washed out immediately with copious amounts of water, 'irrigate, irrigate, irrigate':
- ensure it is safe to approach: put on gloves if available, ventilate the area to disperse fumes and if possible seal the chemical container; it may be necessary to move the casualty
- irrigate the casualty's affected eye with running cold water for at least 10 minutes (Fig. 16.1) (an eye irrigator or a glass may also be used to

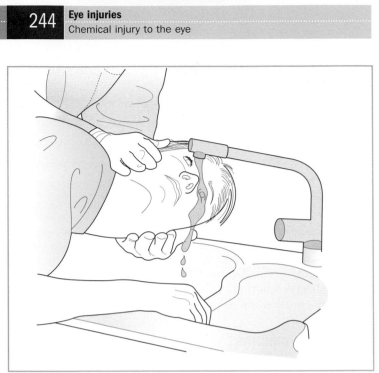

Figure 16.1 Chemical injury to the eye: irrigate the eye, ensuring the water drains away from the face and not into the unaffected eye

pour water over the eye); it may be necessary to prise the eyelids open if there are closed tight in a spasm of pain

- ensure that the eyelid is thoroughly irrigated both inside and out
- take care not to allow contaminated water to splash into the unaffected eye
- apply a sterile eye pad or a clean, non-fluffy pad over the injured eye
- arrange urgent transfer to an Accident & Emergency Department
- identify the chemical if possible
- ask the casualty to keep the uninjured eye still because movement of this will also result in movement of the injured eye which could aggravate the injury
(St John Ambulance, 2002).

CS gas injury

CS gas or 'tear gas' is a solvent spray used by the police for riot control and self-protection. It is sometimes used by unauthorised personnel as an assault weapon.

Effects on the casualty

Effects of CS spray on the casualty include:
- lachrymation
- uncontrolled sneezing and coughing
- burning sensation on the skin and in the throat
- chest tightness
- vomiting
  (Wyatt et al, 2004).

The effects usually wear off within 10–15 minutes, sometimes longer if the spray was used in a confined space.

Treatment

- If possible ensure your own protection from the CS spray
- Escort the casualty to a well-ventilated area
- Reassure the casualty that the symptoms will soon resolve
- If the casualty's eyes are painful, fan them to speed up the vaporisation of the CS chemical; this is preferable to eye irrigation (the standard treatment for chemicals in the eye), which can prolong the burning sensation
- Discourage the casualty from rubbing the eyes
- Arrange transfer to hospital if there is significant exposure to CS spray at close quarters

Penetrating eye injury

A penetrating eye injury is not always obvious and can easily be missed. Any history of a high velocity injury, e.g. use of hammer and chisel, should increase suspicion of a penetrating eye injury.

Treatment

If there is a suspected penetrating eye injury or if one is clearly evident:

* apply a sterile eye pad or a clean, non-fluffy pad over the injured eye to protect it from any pressure (Fig. 16.2)

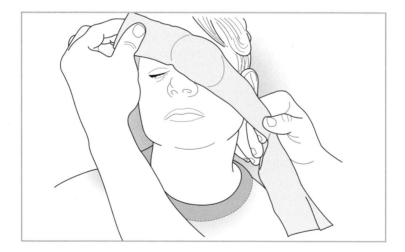

Figure 16.2 Penetrating eye injury: apply a sterile eye pad or a clean, non-fluffy pad over the injured eye to protect it from any pressure

- ask the casualty to keep the uninjured eye still because movement of this will also result in movement of the injured eye which could aggravate the injury

- arrange transfer to an Accident & Emergency Department or a specialist eye unit

- never manipulate and attempt to remove embedded objects, e.g. a dart.

All penetrating eye injuries should receive immediate specialist ophthalmic management without delay

Conclusion

Eye injuries can be very irritating and painful for the casualty. Some can potentially be serious. This chapter has provided an overview to the first aid treatment of eye injuries.

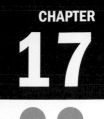

CHAPTER 17

Ear, nose and throat problems

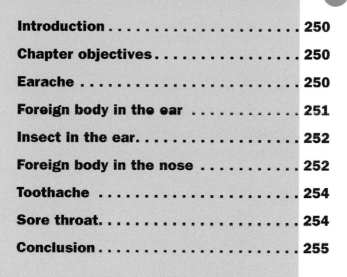

Ear, nose and throat problems

Introduction

Although problems affecting the ear, nose and throat are usually minor, it is important to be aware that, sometimes, serious complications can occur, e.g. repeated ear infections can cause deafness.

The aim of the chapter is to understand the first aid treatment for ear, nose and throat problems.

Chapter objectives

At the end of the chapter the reader will be able to discuss the first aid treatment for:

- **Earache**

- **Foreign body in the ear**

- **Foreign body in the nose**

- **Toothache**

- **Sore throat**

Earache

Earache is usually caused by infection. Young children in particular are prone to middle ear infections because their eustachian tubes can easily become blocked. Sometimes earache is the main presenting symptom of pathology from structures other than the ear, e.g. teeth (abscess) and throat (tonsillitis).

Treatment

- The casualty may wish to take two paracetamol tablets (1 g dose in adults)
- Offer the casualty a source of heat to hold against the ear, e.g. hot water bottle wrapped up in a towel (Fig. 17.1)
- Ensure the casualty is well supported with propped up pillows (lying flat may exacerbate the pain)
- Advise the casualty to see his GP if the pain does not resolve

Foreign body in the ear

A foreign body in the ear is usually encountered in children (intentional insertion), but sometimes is also seen in adults, e.g. end of cotton bud. The casualty may require ENT referral.

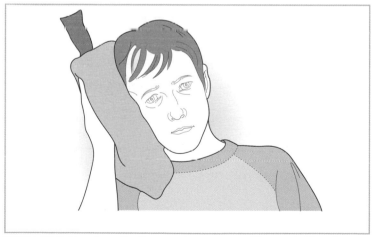

Figure 17.1 Earache: offer the casualty a source of heat to hold against the ear, e.g. hot water bottle wrapped in a towel

Signs and symptoms

Signs and symptoms may include:
• pain and deafness in the one ear
• discharge from the affected ear.

Treatment

• Ask the casualty to turn the head so that the ear with the foreign body is facing the floor: the influence of gravity may dislodge the foreign body

• Do not try physically to remove the foreign body, as this may result in it being pushed further into the ear

• Arrange for transport to an Accident & Emergency Department

Insect in the ear

An insect, such as a fly, trapped in the ear is quite common. The casualty may complain of an irritating buzzing in one ear. To remove the insect, a suggested technique is to:
• ask the casualty to sit down
• ask the casualty to position the head on the side with the affected ear facing upwards
• gently pour tepid water into the ear to drown the insect and flood it out (Fig. 17.2)
• if this fails, arrange for transport to an Accident & Emergency Department.

Foreign body in the nose

A foreign body in the nose is usually inserted intentionally by a child and is often visible. It can block the nose and cause infection. Unilateral purulent nasal discharge usually indicates the presence of a foreign body in the nose.

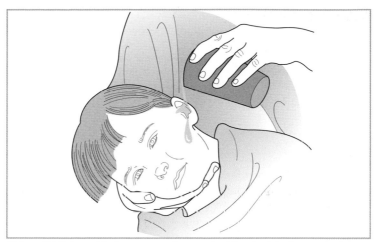

Figure 17.2 Insect in the ear: gently pour tepid water into the ear to drown the insect and flood it out

Signs and symptoms

- Breathing through the nose may be difficult and noisy
- Nasal swelling
- Purulent discharge

Treatment

- Do not try to remove the foreign body, as this may result in it being pushed further into the nose
- Ask the child to blow the nose at the same time as occluding the unaffected nostril
- Arrange for transport to an Accident & Emergency Department

Toothache

Toothache is normally caused by a decaying tooth. If the pain is throbbing in nature, this suggests infection and urgent dental treatment is required. An untreated tooth abscess can be life-threatening.

Treatment

- To help relieve the pain, the casualty may wish to take two paracetamol tablets (1 g dose in adults); cotton wool soaked in oil of cloves pressed against the affected tooth may provide some pain relief
- The casualty may find it more comfortable to sit up, well supported with pillows (lying flat may exacerbate the pain)
- Advise the casualty to contact his dentist

Sore throat

A sore throat is often the first sign that the casualty is developing a cough or cold. It is usually caused by a viral infection and will resolve without treatment after a couple of days.

Treatment

- Encourage the casualty to drink plenty of cool drinks; these help to relieve pain and stop the throat becoming dry
- To help relieve the pain, the casualty may wish to take two paracetamol tablets (1 g dose in adults)

Tonsillitis

If the casualty develops tonsillitis, medical referral will be required. Antibiotics will be prescribed; symptomatic treatment includes bed rest, a liquid diet and soluble aspirin to relieve pain.

Conclusion

This chapter has highlighted the first aid treatment for ear, nose and throat problems, including earache, foreign body in the ear, foreign body in the nose, toothache and sore throat.

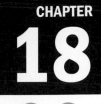

CHAPTER

18

Poisoning, stings and bites

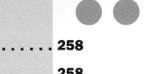

Poisoning, stings and bites

Introduction

Poisoning is usually unintentional, e.g. following exposure to a toxic substance such as carbon monoxide, or can be intentional, e.g. attempted suicide. First aid treatment is usually supportive, particularly with attention to the maintenance of a clear airway (altered conscious level is common). In the UK, insect stings are usually only minor, but occasionally they can cause anaphylaxis. Animal and human bites always require medical attention because of the infection risk.

Chapter objectives
At the end of the chapter the reader will be able to discuss the

- **General treatment measures for poisoning**

- **Treatment for carbon monoxide poisoning**

- **Treatment for bee and wasp stings**

- **Treatment for human and animal bites**

- **Treatment for snake bites**

General treatment measures for poisoning

Whether accidental or intentional, poisoning is a common problem encountered in the pre-hospital environment. Acute poisoning accounts for 100 000 hospital admissions in England and Wales.

Poisoning, stings and bites
General treatment measures for poisoning
259

Poisoning is a leading cause of cardiac arrest in the <40 years age group (Resuscitation Council (UK), 2000). With some poisoning agents, cardiac arrest results from direct cardiotoxicity while with others it is secondary to respiratory arrest caused by CNS depression or aspiration of gastric contents.

Wherever possible the constituents of the ingested substance should be accurately identified. Some idea of the maximum amount of the substance that could have been ingested can be determined by comparing the number of tablets, or volume of liquid remaining, with details on the packaging.

In respect of drug overdose, the following information would be helpful for the emergency services:
- substance(s) ingested
- how much was ingested
- timing
- by what route
- alcohol taken as well
- history of drug abuse
- past medical history.

Treatment

- Ensure it is safe to approach; in some poisoning situations, e.g. industrial accident, it may be necessary to move the casualty from the area before treatment can begin
- If possible, prevent further exposure or absorption of the poison
- If possible identify the poison
- Monitor the casualty's vital signs, in particular the conscious level; the management of most acute poisoning is supportive, e.g. if the casualty is unconscious, place in the recovery position
- Send tablets and empty bottles to the hospital
- In the case of ingestion of bleach, fluids should be encouraged, particularly milk

Carbon monoxide poisoning

Carbon monoxide is a colourless, odourless and tasteless gas that is very toxic when inhaled. Common sources of carbon monoxide include most types of smoke, car exhaust fumes, defective gas or paraffin heaters and blocked chimney flues.

Effects

Carbon monoxide poisoning causes tissue hypoxia by:
- interrupting electron transport in mitochondria
- reducing tissue oxygenation by competing with O2 for binding with haemoglobin
  (Ramrakha & Moore, 2004).

Susceptibility to carbon monoxide is increased if there is anaemia, increased metabolic rate, e.g. in children or ischaemic heart disease.

Signs and symptoms

Signs and symptoms of carbon monoxide poisoning include:
- signs of hypoxia without cyanosis
- COHb <30%: headaches and dizziness
- COHb 50–60%: syncope, tachypnoea, tachycardia and seizures
- COHb >60%: risk of cardiopulmonary arrest
  (Ramrakha & Moore, 2004).

The so-called 'classic' feature of cherry red mucous membranes is a rarely seen, completely unreliable clinical sign

Treatment

- If possible, evacuate the casualty into fresh air
- Loosen any tight clothing worn by the casualty

Poisoning, stings and bites
Human and animal bites
261

- Check the casualty's conscious level. If unconscious, but breathing, place in the recovery position. If not breathing, start resuscitation
- Ensure the emergency services are alerted immediately

The casualty will require high concentrations of inspired oxygen. Pulse oximetry will be unreliable and misleading. If the casualty has carboxyhaemoglobinaemia, hyperbaric oxygen may be required, particularly if the casualty has been unconscious, has cardiac or neurological symptoms or is pregnant.

Bee and wasp stings

Bee and wasp stings are very painful, can cause local infection and occasionally can cause anaphylaxis.

Treatment

- Help the casualty to sit down
- Scrape any insect parts off the skin, but do not squeeze them as this allegedly increases envenomation (AHA & ILCOR, 2000)
- If possible, raise the affected part
- Apply a cold press or ice to help relieve the pain
- Advise the casualty to seek medical help if the pain and swelling persist
- If casualty displays signs of anaphylaxis alert the emergency services; assist with the use of adrenaline (epinephrine) auto-injector device if there is one (see Chapter 7)

Human and animal bites

Human and animal bites can be serious. All bites carry a risk of infection including tetanus and rabies, particularly if the bite occurred abroad. There are approximately 30–40 tetanus cases in the UK each year; *Clostridium tetani* spores are commonly found in soil and animal faeces.

If the skin is broken, prompt first aid is required to minimise the risk of infection. The need for anti-tetanus prophylaxis should also be considered.

Anti-tetanus prophylaxis

Anti-tetanus prophylaxis will depend upon the tetanus status of the casualty and whether the wound is 'clean' or 'tetanus-prone', e.g. puncture wound, animal bite.

Treatment

- Thoroughly wash the wound using warm soapy water
- Arrange transfer to hospital if the wound is large or deep, or if anti-tetanus prophylaxis is required. If a human, dog or cat bite causes a break in the skin, antibiotics will be prescribed.

Snake bite

The adder, the only native venomous snake in the UK, has a distinguishing dark zig-zag pattern marking on its back. Although its bite is rarely fatal, it will certainly be frightening for the casualty. The bite will result in two puncture holes, 1 cm apart; initially there will be local pain and swelling, abdominal pain, vomiting and diarrhoea, and shock may follow.

Treatment

- Help the casualty to lie down
- Alert the emergency services
- Rest and bandage the injured part to slow down lymphatic flow
- Note the appearance of the snake and pass this information on to the emergency services

- Do not apply a tourniquet or attempt to suck the venom out (St John Ambulance, 2002)

Conclusion

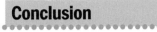

First aid treatment for poisoning is usually supportive, particularly with attention to the maintenance of a clear airway. Insect stings are usually only minor, but occasionally they can cause anaphylaxis. Animal and human bites will require medical attention because of the infection risk.

Childhood illnesses

Childhood illnesses

Introduction

Children are not small adults. They differ from adults anatomically, physiologically, emotionally and in terms of the range of diseases they are susceptible to. When infants and children are ill, they can deteriorate alarmingly quickly. The importance of the early recognition of serious illness has been discussed in Chapter 5. It is also important not to forget the child's parents. They may be very anxious and upset and will therefore also need help and support.

The aim of this chapter is understand the first aid treatment of common childhood illnesses.

Chapter objectives
At the end of the chapter the reader will be able to discuss the first aid treatment for:

- **Bacterial meningitis**
- **Croup**
- **Epiglottitis**
- **Bronchiolitis**
- **Asthma**
- **Seizures**
- **Poisoning**

Bacterial meningitis

Meningitis is an important medical emergency demanding early diagnosis and prompt treatment. Bacterial meningitis is often caused by *Neisseria meningitidis* (meningococcus) or by pneumococcal bacteria, the latter generally only affecting children <2 years of age.

Widespread *Haemophilus influenzae* B (Hib) vaccination has led to a reduction in the incidence of *Haemophilus influenzae* infection by over 90% (Meningitis Research Foundation, 2005). Hib meningitis is now rare in countries that use the vaccine, but still very common in countries that do not.

In newborn babies, the commonest cause of meningitis is Group B streptococcal bacteria; 90% of babies infected with this disease survive with most having no significant long-term effects (Meningitis Research Foundation, 2005).

Signs and symptoms

<4 years of age

In this age group bacterial meningitis can be difficult to diagnose; neck rigidity, photophobia, headache and vomiting are usually absent. Signs and symptoms of meningitis are primarily those of increased intracranial pressure:

- coma
- drowsiness (usually lack of eye contact)
- high-pitched cry or irritability that cannot be easily soothed by the parent
- poor feeding
- pyrexia of unknown cause
- convulsions with or without fever
- purpuric rash
- apnoeic or cyanotic attacks

Although, in infants, a bulging fontanelle is an advanced sign of meningitis, this late and serious sign will be masked if vomiting and fever have led to dehydration.

4 years of age and above

In this age group, the classic signs of meningitis are more likely to be present:

- headache
- vomiting
- pyrexia
- neck rigidity
- photophobia
  (ALSG, 2005).

The child may present with coma or convulsions. The presence of a purpuric rash in an ill child is almost certainly due to meningococcal infection; immediate treatment will be required, and urgent transfer to hospital should be arranged. Viral meningitis is usually mild and medical treatment is often not required (Meningitis Research Foundation, 2005).

Tumbler test: press a glass tumbler against the rash: the rash will be visible through the glass and does not fade (Fig. 19.1).

Treatment

- If meningitis is suspected, seek medical help immediately; if the GP cannot be contacted or if he is going to be delayed, alert the emergency services
- While awaiting help, reassure the child
- Consider paracetamol for pyrexia

Croup

Croup, or laryngotracheobronchitis, is a common childhood illness most often caused by a viral infection. It is usually a benign, self-limiting disease, but can result in life-threatening upper airway obstruction.

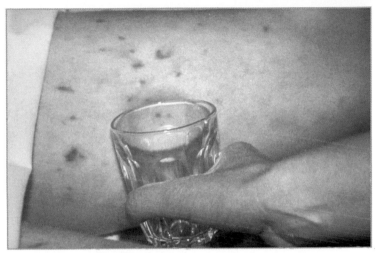

Figure 19.1 The glass test: the rash does not fade under pressure and will still be visible when the side of the clear glass is pressed firmly against the skin. ® Meningitis Research Foundation. Reproduced with kind permission of Meningitis Research Foundation

Acute viral laryngotracheobronchitis (viral croup) is the commonest form of croup, accounting for >95% of laryngotracheal infections (ALSG, 2005). The peak age incidence of viral croup is 1–2 years, with most hospital admissions occurring in children aged 6 months to 5 years (ALSG, 2005).

In an awake, alert child, obstruction of the upper airway is usually due to croup, with inflammation, oedema, and narrowing of the larynx, trachea and bronchioles. It is important to exclude the potentially fatal infection, epiglottitis.

Signs and symptoms

Most children with croup will have had several days of cold symptoms and fever. The symptoms of croup, which often start and are worse at night, may include:

- inspiratory stridor
- barking cough
- hoarseness
- variable degrees of respiratory distress
- fever
  (Resuscitation Council UK, 2003).

Treatment

Most children with croup can be managed at home. The following can be helpful:

- Sitting the child upright, on the parent's knee supporting the back
- Carrying the child in cool fresh air
- Encouraging plenty of cool drinks (to prevent dehydration)
- Administering paracetamol suspension, e.g. Calpol, if the child is pyrexial
- Removing the child's clothing (if the room is warm)
- Avoiding smoky environments
- Reassuring the child and try to keep the child calm; try not to frighten or agitate the child
- Creating a humid atmosphere at night, e.g. hang a wet towel on the radiator in the child's bedroom
  (St John Ambulance, 2002; Nursing Times, 2005).

Children with respiratory distress may need hospital admission and supportive treatment. Steroids, e.g. dexamethasone orally or IV, can help relieve the symptoms faster and may lead to a reduction in hospital stay. Very occasionally, a child with croup will require intubation due to a combination of exhaustion and respiratory failure resulting from upper airway obstruction. Cardiopulmonary arrest can complicate croup, particularly in infants.

Epiglottitis

Epiglottitis (inflammation of the epiglottis) is now very rare due to the widespread *Haemophilus influenzae* B (Hib) vaccination. However, it is still encountered (unimmunised children and failed vaccination). It is predominantly seen in children aged 1–6 years, but can occur in infants and adults (ALSG, 2005).

The onset is usually sudden and the resultant swelling of the epiglottis and the surrounding tissues can rapidly lead to life-threatening airway obstruction.

Signs and symptoms

- Respiratory difficulty
- High fever (>39°C)
- Lethargy
- Soft inspiratory stridor
- Hoarseness
- Pallor
- Absent or minimal cough
- Drooling at the mouth (reluctance or inability to swallow)
  (Resuscitation Council UK, 2003)

Treatment

Urgent transfer to hospital should be arranged. The child will need the airway secured and antibiotic therapy (usually cefotaxime) started (ALSG, 2005).

While waiting for the emergency services:
- leave the child with the parent in a comfortable position. Do not move the child, upset the child or lie the child down; this could lead to airway obstruction

- continually monitor the child's vital signs
- do not attempt to look down the child's throat; the child may start crying which could aggravate the situation.

Bronchiolitis

Bronchiolitis is the commonest serious respiratory condition in childhood: it occurs in 10% of infants and 2–3% require hospital admission each year (ALSG, 2005). Ninety per cent of cases are in infants aged 1–9 months and it is rare in children >1 year of age. Often caused by the respiratory syncytial virus, it is widespread in the winter months.

Infants are particularly vulnerable because of the small size of their airways, high resistance to airflow and poor airway clearance. Risk factors for respiratory failure in infants with bronchiolitis include premature birth, <2 months of age, underlying lung disease, congenital heart disease, and immunodeficiency. Problems with feeding associated with increasing dyspnoea are often the reason for hospital admission.

Signs and symptoms

Signs and symptoms may include:
- Sharp, dry cough
- Tachycardia
- Fever
- Subcostal and intercostal recession
- Tachypnoea
- Wheeze
- Poor feeding
  (American Academy of Pediatrics, 2000)

Treatment

For mild bronchiolitis, the infant will probably be cared for at home. The following treatment is recommended:
- administer plenty of fluids
- offer paracetamol suspension if the infant is pyrexial
- provide small feeds regularly
- if there is thick mucus in the lungs, slap the infant's back to loosen it.

There is no specific treatment for bronchiolitis; management is supportive. Bronchodilators, adrenaline (epinephrine) and corticosteroids are often used, though this is controversial (Scarphone, 2005). Two per cent of infants admitted to hospital require mechanical ventilation (ALSG, 2005).

Recurrent apnoea can complicate bronchiolitis, particularly those born prematurely. Close monitoring of the infant's vital signs is essential.

Acute asthma

Many asthma-related deaths are preventable

The management of acute asthma has been discussed in Chapter 8. Some important considerations related to severe asthma in children will now be discussed.

Assessment

In acute asthma the following in particular should be assessed:
- Pulse rate
- Respiratory rate, together with degree of breathlessness
- Use of accessory muscles
- Severity of wheeze

- Degree of agitation and conscious level (British Thoracic Society & Scottish Intercollegiate Guidelines Network (BTS & SIGN), 2004).

Signs of acute severe asthma

- Child is too breathless to talk or to feed
- Heart rate >120 in children >5 years of age (>130 in children 2–5 years of age)
- Respiratory rate >30/minute in children >5 years of age (>50/minute in children 2–5 years of age) (BTS & SIGN, 2004)

Some children with acute severe asthma do not appear distressed

Signs of life-threatening asthma

- Silent chest
- Cyanosis
- Poor respiratory effort
- Falling heart rate
- Exhaustion
- Confusion
- Coma (BTS & SIGN, 2004)

Treatment

- Assess the child's respiratory function.
- Leave the child with the parent; normally the child will adopt his own position to help breathing
- If available, consult the child's individual action plan in the event of an asthma attack

- Encourage the parents to administer the prescribed relief inhaler; this will probably be via a spacer device with or without facemask (Fig. 19.2)
- Monitor the child's vital signs, particularly respiratory rate, heart rate and conscious level

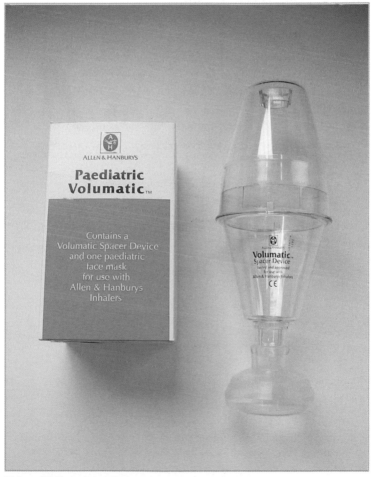

Figure 19.2 Acute asthma: spacer device

- In an older child, record peak expiratory flow (PEF) if he has a PEF meter (see Fig. 8.3); document the result

- Reassure the child and parents; an acute attack of asthma is frightening and hospital transfer may increase anxiety and exacerbate symptoms; reassurance that treatment is available to relieve the attack is an important aspect of care

- Ensure the emergency services have been alerted (see below)

Indications for hospital admission

Asthma has been classified into moderate, severe and life-threatening (BTS & SIGN, 2005) (see Fig. 8.1). For moderate, severe and life-threatening asthma, the following is recommended.

Moderate asthma: treat at home and assess response to treatment.

Severe asthma: immediate transfer to hospital should be arranged if the casualty is not responding to treatment after 15 minutes.

Life-threatening asthma: immediate transfer to hospital should be arranged.

Factors lowering the threshold for hospital admission include:
- afternoon or night attack

- recent hospital admission

- previous severe attack

- concern regarding social circumstances or ability to cope at home (BTS & SIGN, 2005)

Seizures

Seizures are common in children; 5% will have at least one seizure by the age of 6 years (American Academy of Pediatrics, 2000). Prolonged seizures can have profound adverse effects including an increase in cerebral metabolic rate, peripheral vasoconstriction, a decrease in systemic blood pressure, a fall in cerebral blood flow and the accumulation of lactic acid which can lead to cell death, oedema and a rise in intracerebral pressure.

Most paediatric seizures are caused by fever (febrile seizures); up to 5% of children with febrile seizures present with status epilepticus (ALSG, 2005). Status epilepticus can be fatal (4%) and death can be caused by a number of factors, including airway obstruction, hypoxia and aspiration of vomit (ALSG, 2005). Febrile seizures are usually brief (<15 minutes) and rarely cause cerebral injury.

Infants <6 months presenting with first-time seizures may have significant underlying pathology, which could include immediately life-threatening conditions, and may look deceptively well on initial evaluation.

Causes

- Fever: accounts for 30% of paediatric seizures (febrile seizures)
- Hypoxia
- Hypoglycaemia
- Infection
- Head injury
- Cerebral insult
- Idiopathic

Signs and symptoms

- Violent muscle twitching, clenched fists and an arched back – classic signs of a seizure
- Fever and associated hot, flushed skin may be present
- Twitching of the face
- Fixed, upturned or squinting eyes
- Loss of or impaired consciousness

- Breath-holding
- Red 'puffy' face and neck
- Drooling at the mouth (St John Ambulance, 2002)

Treatment

- Alert the emergency services
- Prevent injury to the child
- Observe for neck rigidity in a child and a full fontanelle in an infant; their presence suggests meningitis
- If fever present: remove clothes (undress down to the underpants) and ensure a good supply of cool, fresh air, taking care not to overcool the child
- Assess and if necessary support airway, breathing and circulation – upper airway obstruction can be caused by secretions or tongue hyotonia. Respiratory arrest can occur due to depression of the central nervous system, particularly if the child is taking anti-epileptic medication
- Take a history: specific points include current fever, recent trauma, history of epilepsy, ingestion of poison, known illnesses and last meal

Observe for neck rigidity in a child and a full fontanelle in an infant; their presence suggests meningitis

Poisoning

Infants and children account for most admissions to A & E departments with poisoning, accounting for up to 70% of all toxic exposures.

Eighty per cent of poisoning in children occurs in the <5 year age group; usually only one poison is involved and the exposure is usually small and unintentional. However, in school-aged children and adolescents, toxic exposures are often intentional, either for recreation or as a suicide attempt or gesture.

Nervous system depression is a common symptom of poisoning; it may lead to airway compromise, respiratory failure or aspiration.

History is the best tool for assessment in paediatric poisoning and is considered to be usually more accurate than physical examination when trying to establish the specific type of toxic exposure. It is helpful if the agent can be identified, together with the amount involved, and when the exposure occurred.

Identifying the poison

Wherever possible the constituents of the ingested substance should be accurately identified. Some idea of the maximum amount of the substance that could have been ingested can be determined by comparing the number of tablets, or volume of liquid remaining, with details on the packaging. It is important not to overlook the involvement of other children in a poisoning incident.

Treatment

- Ensure the safety of both the child and the rescuer
- Alert the emergency services
- Monitor the child's vital signs as appropriate
- Prevent further exposure to the poison
- If the child is unconscious, but breathing, place in the recovery position
- Monitor the child's conscious level
- In the case of ingestion of bleach, fluids should be encouraged, particularly milk

Conclusion

Children differ to adults anatomically, physiologically, emotionally and in terms of the range of diseases they are susceptible to. When they are ill, they can deteriorate alarmingly quickly. The chapter has provided an overview of the first aid treatment of common childhood illnesses.

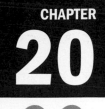
Dressings, bandages and slings

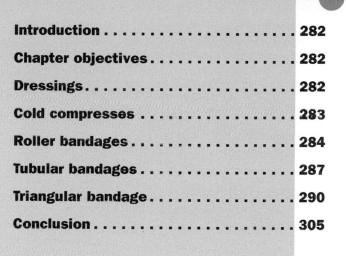

Dressings, bandages and slings

Introduction

Bandages can be used to secure dressings, control bleeding, immobilise and support limbs and reduce swelling. There are three types of bandages: roller, tubular and triangular. Triangular bandages are often used to form slings.

Most of the information in this chapter is based on recommendations from the voluntary first aid societies – St John Ambulance, 2002 and British Red Cross, 2003.

At the end of the chapter the reader will be able to understand the principles of the use of dressings, bandages and slings.

Chapter objectives
At the end of the chapter the reader will be able to describe how to use

- **Dressings**
- **Cold compresses**
- **Roller bandages**
- **Tubular bandages**
- **Triangular bandages**

Dressings

Applying a dressing will help to keep the wound dry and will provide some degree of protection. There are many different types of wound dressings currently available. Some important points to consider when using a dressing:

- ensure the dressing is large enough to fit comfortably over the wound
- use a sterile dressing if possible; if not available, a clean non-fluffy dressing will suffice
- when applying the dressing, ensure to handle it using its edges
- use adhesive dressings (plasters) for small cuts and grazes (ensure the casualty is not allergic to plaster)
- do not remove a dressing if the wound continues to bleed through it: apply additional dressing(s) on top.

Improvised dressings (clean and non-fluffy) include sanitary towels, tea-towels and torn-up sheets.

Cold compresses

The application of a cold compress can help to reduce swelling and relieve pain. It can be particularly helpful for treating bruising and sprains. There are two methods of applying a cold press: a cold pad or an ice pack.

Cold pad

- Soak a pad (towel, flannel or similar) in cold water; then wring it out
- Apply the pad firmly over the injury
- Regularly re-soak the pad in cold water to keep it cold

Ice pack

- Partly fill up a plastic bag with ice cubes and then seal it (a bag of frozen vegetables will suffice)
- Wrap it up in a dry cloth or towel
- Apply the pad firmly over the injury
- Replace the bag as required

Do not apply ice directly onto the skin, as it may burn it

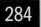

Roller bandages

Roller bandages are used to support limbs, secure dressings and, by applying pressure, to control bleeding. They are made of cotton, gauze, linen or elasticated fabric.

Types

Roller bandages are available in three types.

Open-weave: allow ventilation and are used to secure dressings; cannot be used to exert pressure or support limbs.

Elasticated: mould to the shape of the body and are used to support soft tissue injuries and secure dressings.

Crepe: provide firm support to injured joints.

The tip of the bandage is called the 'tail' and the rolled up part the 'head' (Fig. 20.1). The correct sizes of bandages to be used in adults for different use are detailed in Box 20.1.

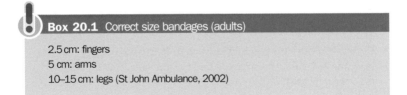

Box 20.1 Correct size bandages (adults)

2.5 cm: fingers
5 cm: arms
10–15 cm: legs (St John Ambulance, 2002)

Standard application of a roller bandage

- Explain the procedure to the casualty
- Select an appropriate bandage and the correct size (Box 20.1)
- Adopt a position in front of the casualty, on the injured side

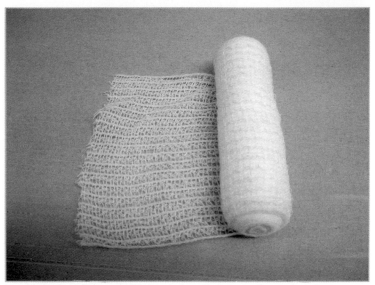

Figure 20.1 Roller bandage: the tip is called the 'tail' and the rolled up part the 'head'

- Ensure the injured part is supported in the position it needs to remain in after bandaging
- Ensure the 'head' of the bandage is uppermost
- Place the 'tail' below the injury and start bandaging from the inside to the outside of the limb, beginning from the bottom of the limb and working upwards (Fig. 20.2)
- Ensure that the bandage is applied firmly
- Starting with two overlapping turns to secure the 'tail', roll the bandage around the limb, ensuring each new turn covers half of the previous turn
- Finish with two overlapping turns and secure the bandage (e.g. adhesive tape, bandage clip, safety pin or 'tuck' in loose end)
- Apply another bandage if required

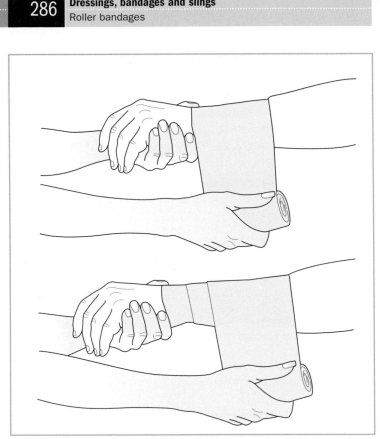

Figure 20.2 Application of the roller bandage: place the 'tail' below the injury and start bandaging from the inside to the outside of the limb, beginning from the bottom of the limb and working upwards

- Check the circulation (e.g. pulses, colour, capillary refill) distal to the bandage: roller bandages can impede circulation
- If the bandage is impeding circulation, unroll it and reapply, ensuring it is slightly looser and then reassess circulation
- Advise the casualty how to monitor the circulation distal to the bandage: swelling could result in the bandage becoming tighter

Application of a knee or elbow bandage

- Explain the procedure to the casualty
- Support the joint, in a slightly flexed position if possible (will help ensure the bandage remains secure)
- Position the 'tail' on the inside of the joint and start with two overlapping turns to secure it
- Then apply the bandage in 'figure of eight' turns
- Finish with two overlapping turns, secure the bandage and check the circulation etc (as above)

Application of a hand and foot bandage

Procedure for the application of hand bandage

- Explain the procedure to the casualty
- Position the 'tail' on the inner wrist and start with two overlapping turns to secure it
- Then apply the bandage in 'figure of eight' turns, ensuring the bandage does not go beyond the nail on the little finger and that the thumb remains free (Fig. 20.3)
- Ensure that each new turn covers half of the previous turn
- Finish with two overlapping turns, secure the bandage and check the circulation (as above)

This procedure can also be used for the application of a foot bandage, but start instead at the base of the big toe and leave the heel unbandaged.

Tubular bandages

Tubular bandages, made of seamless tubular fabric, are useful for holding dressings in place, but are cannot be used to control bleeding because they do not exert sufficient pressure. There are two types.

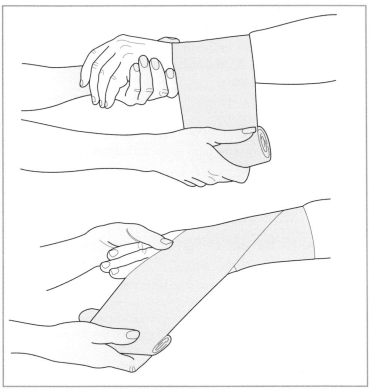

Figure 20.3 Bandaging: figure of 8

Tubular gauze: for covering a finger or toe (comes with an applicator).

Tubular elasticated bandage: for supporting injured joints.

Application of a tubular gauze bandage

- Explain the procedure to the casualty

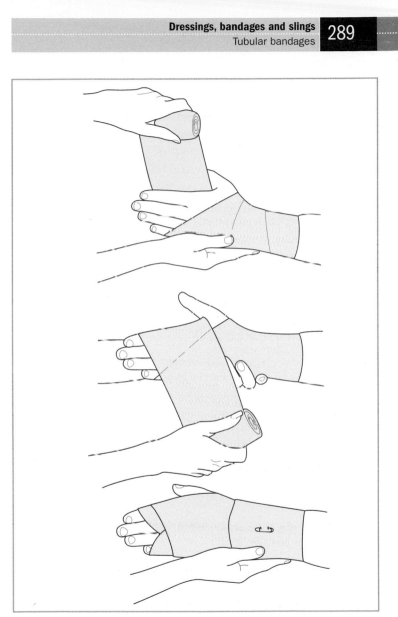

Figure 20.3 *(cont'd)*

- Slide a piece of tubular gauze bandage, equal to 2–3 times the length of the casualty's finger, onto the applicator
- Carefully slide the applicator over the casualty's finger
- While holding the bandage at the base of the casualty's finger, withdraw the applicator just beyond the finger-tip
- Twist the applicator and bandage around twice (Fig. 20.4)
- Carefully slide the applicator back over the casualty's finger to apply a second layer
- Remove the applicator altogether once all the bandage has been applied
- Secure the bandage at the base of the finger with some tape
- Monitor the circulation in the finger: if the casualty complains that the finger feels cold or is tingling, remove the bandage and re-apply it more loosely

Triangular bandage

A triangular bandage can broad-folded, narrow-folded or it can also be opened and used as a scalp bandage or to form a sling.

Broad-fold bandage

A broad-fold bandage can be used to immobilise and support an injured limb, secure a dressing or stabilise a splint. To make a broad fold bandage:

1 open out the bandage and place it on a flat, dry and clean surface (Fig. 20.5A)
2 fold the bandage horizontally in half, so that the point touches the centre of the base (Fig. 20.5B)
3 fold the bandage horizontally in half again (Fig. 20.5C).

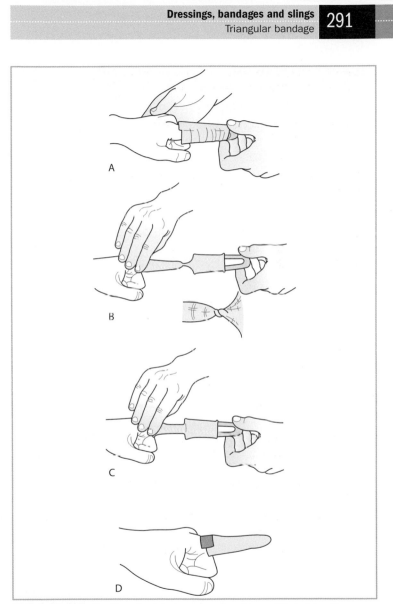

Figure 20.4 Application of a tubular gauze bandage: while holding the bandage at the base of the casualty's finger, withdraw the applicator just beyond the finger-tip; twist the applicator and bandage around twice

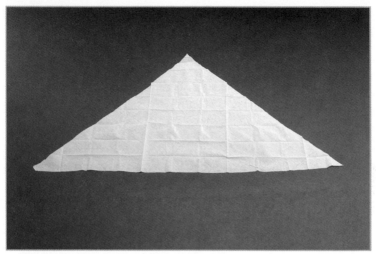

Figure 20.5A Open out the triangular bandage

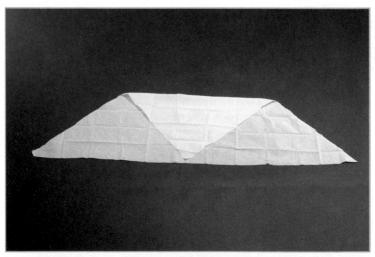

Figure 20.5B Fold the bandage horizontally in half, so that the point touches the centre of the base

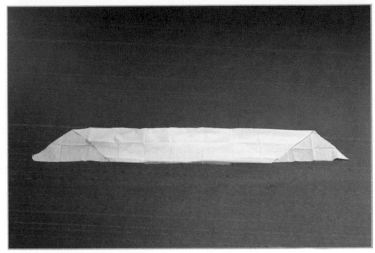

Figure 20.5C Fold the bandage horizontally in half again

Narrow-fold bandage

A narrow-fold bandage can be used to immobilise and support a foot or ankle, or to secure a dressing. To make a narrow-fold bandage:

1 open out the bandage and place it on a flat, dry and clean surface

2 fold the bandage horizontally in half, so that the point touches the centre of the base

3 fold the bandage horizontally in half again

4 fold the bandage horizontally in half again.

Scalp bandage

1 Ensure the casualty is sitting down and the necessary dressing has been applied to the scalp wound

2 After folding a hem along its base, place the bandage (hem side down) on the casualty's head

3 Grasp the two end 'tails', cross them over one another, bring them round to the casualty's forehead and tie them together (Fig. 20.6)

4 Take the other loose end up and secure on top of the casualty's head

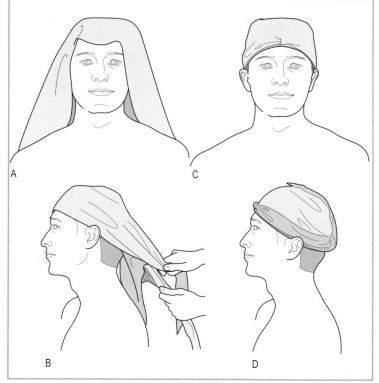

Figure 20.6 Scalp bandage: place the bandage (hem side down) on the casualty's head and grasp the two end 'tails', cross them over one another, bring them round to the casualty's forehead and tie them together

Arm sling

An arm sling can be used to support an injured upper limb and to immobilise an arm if the casualty has a chest injury. It supports the arm horizontally.

1 Ask the casualty to sit down and support the injured arm; the hand on the injured side should be resting slightly above the elbow on the uninjured side (Fig. 20.7A)

2 Open up the triangular bandage and place it on the casualty's chest, sliding it underneath the injured arm; the long straight edge should lie vertically on the uninjured side and the upper tip should be pulled up around the neck and at the shoulder (Fig. 20.7B)

3 Bring the lower tip of the bandage up to meet the upper tip at the shoulder

4 Tie the two tips together in the hollow just above the clavicle using a reef knot; the casualty can now stop supporting the injured arm

5 Fold over the excess bandage at the elbow and secure (Fig. 20.7C)

6 Check and monitor the circulation in the fingers on the injured limb

If a triangular bandage is not available it is possible to improvise an arm sling using either a buttoned up jacket or an unzipped jacket.

- **Jacket with buttons:** place the hand of the injured limb in between the buttons (Fig. 20.8). The hand will then rest on the lower button.
- **Jacket with zip:** unzip the jacket and fold up the jacket over the injured arm and secure it with a safety pin to the top of the jacket (Fig. 20.8).

Elevation sling

An elevation sling can be used to support an injured limb, and at the same time help to reduce pain, swelling and bleeding.

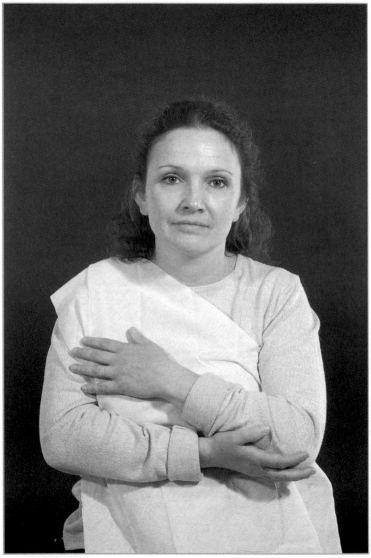

Figure 20.7A Ask the casualty to support the injured arm. Reproduced with permission

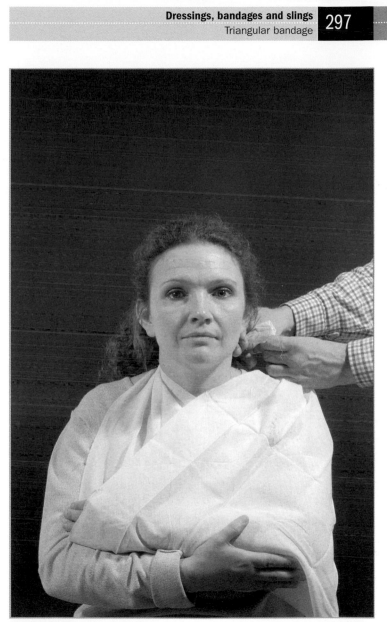

Figure 20.7B Place opened up triangular bandage on the casualty's chest.
Reproduced with permission

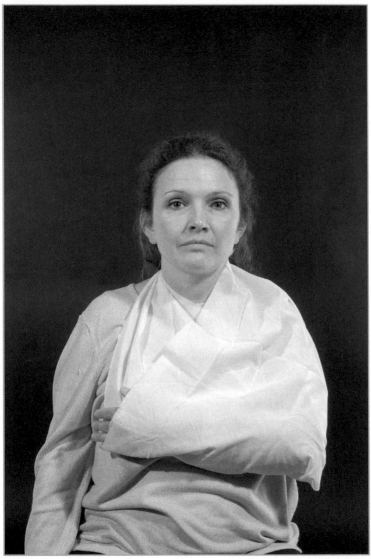

Figure 20.7C Fold over the excess bandage at the elbow and secure. Reproduced with permission

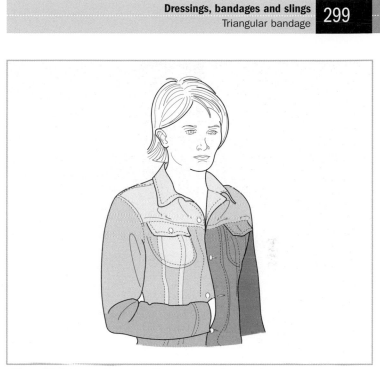

Figure 20.8 Improvised arm slings; using a buttoned up jacket or an unzipped jacket

1 Ask the casualty to sit down and support the injured arm across the chest so that the fingers of the hand on the injured side are touching the clavicle on the uninjured side (Fig. 20.9A)

2 Open up the triangular bandage and place it on the casualty's chest over the injured arm; the long straight edge should lie vertically on the uninjured side and the upper tip should be pulled up over the shoulder (Fig. 20.9B)

3 Grasping the bottom tip, bring it up and tuck it behind the injured limb, through to the casualty's back and up towards the shoulder on the uninjured side

4 Tie the two tips together in the hollow just above the clavicle using a reef knot; the casualty can now stop supporting the injured arm

5 Fold over the excess bandage at the elbow and secure (Fig. 20.9C)

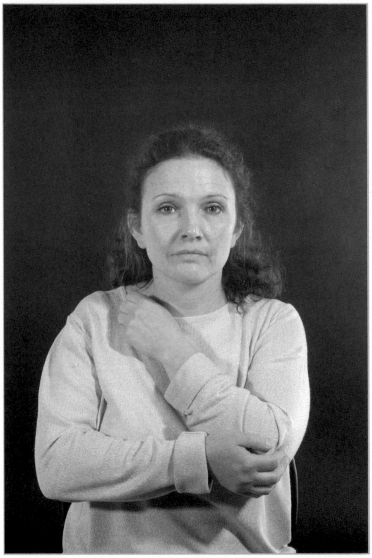

Figure 20.9A Ask the casualty to place the injured arm across the chest.
Reproduced with permission

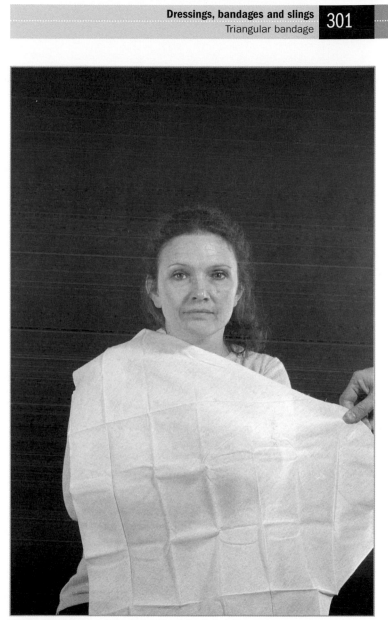

Figure 20.9B Place open the triangular bandage on the casualty's chest.
Reproduced with permission

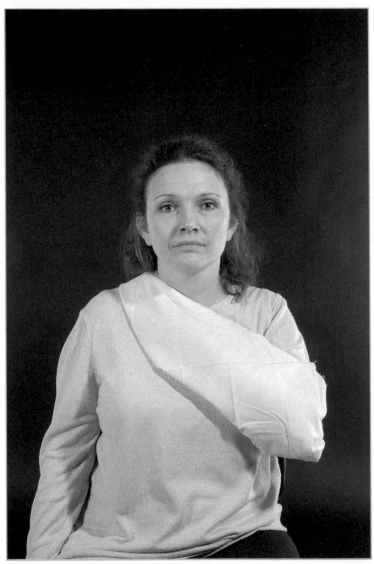

Figure 20.9C Fold over the excess bandage at the elbow and secure.
Reproduced with permission

6 Check and monitor the circulation in the fingers and thumb on the injured limb

If a triangular bandage is not available it is possible to improvise an elevation sling using a long sleeved shirt or a belt/tie/pair of tights.

- Ask the casualty to support the injured arm across the chest so that the fingers of the hand on the injured side are touching the clavicle on the uninjured side; then secure the shirt sleeve to the casualty's shirt using a safety pin (Fig. 20.10A)
- Use belt/tie/pair of tights or similar to make a 'collar and cuff' support: tie the two ends together, place it over the casualty's head and then twist it to produce a loop; place the casualty's hand in the loop (Fig. 20.10B) (monitor circulation in the hand)

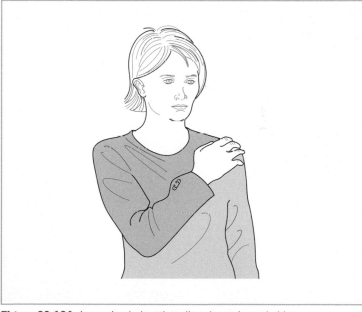

Figure 20.10A Improvised elevation sling: long sleeved shirt

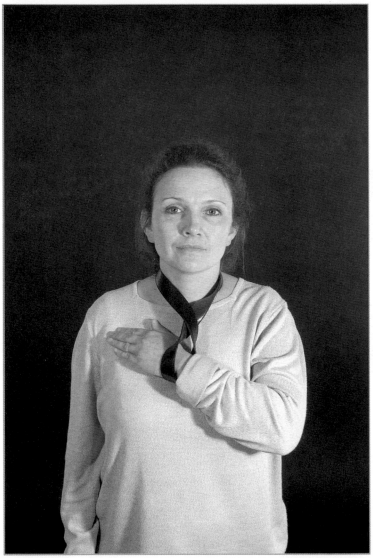

Figure 20.10B Improvised elevation sling: belt/tie/pair of tights or similar to make a 'collar and cuff' support. Reproduced with permission

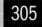

Conclusion

Bandages can be used to secure dressings, control bleeding, immobilise and support limbs and reduce swelling. The principles of the use of dressings, bandages and slings have been described in this chapter. Details of how to improvise have also been discussed.

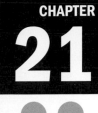

Legal aspects of first aid

CHAPTER 21

Bridgit Dimond

Legal aspects of first aid

Introduction

This chapter attempts to explore the law that relates to the work of the first aider, both as a professional and also as a volunteer. It considers the background to the legal system and then looks at several possible scenarios which may confront those providing first aid and discusses the legal issues that arise. An extended reading list is provided for those interested in further study.

Background to the legal system and the NHS

Legal system

Laws derive from two main sources. First, Acts of Parliament (known as primary legislation) and regulations (known as secondary legislation) or directions from the European Community and, secondly, the decisions in cases decided by the courts (known as the common law, or judge made law or case law). The Assemblies of Scotland, Wales and Northern Ireland have varying law making powers. Primary legislation often gives powers to a minister of the crown to make further more detailed regulations. These are usually drawn up in the form of a statutory instrument which is laid before Parliament for approval or rejection before it comes into force.

Human Rights Act

This Act came into force on 2 October 2000 (in Scotland on devolution) and has three effects:

- All public authorities or organisations carrying out functions of a public nature are required to respect the European Convention of Human Rights which is set out in Schedule 1 to the Act.
- Citizens have a right to bring an action in the courts of the UK if they considered that their human rights, as set out in the Schedule, had been breached by a public authority.
- Judges are required to refer back to Parliament any legislation which they considered to be incompatible with the Articles set out in the European Convention of Human Rights.

One of the most significant changes brought about by this Act is that people no longer have to take their case to Strasbourg for a hearing before the European Courts of Human Rights but can avoid the additional cost and delay and bring the case in UK courts. If a judicial review is sought of a decision which is considered to be in breach of the human rights recognised in the Convention, then legal aid is available for this action.

Of specific significance to first aid care are the following Articles:
- Article 2: the right to life
- Article 3: the right not to be subjected to torture or to inhuman or degrading treatment and punishment
- Article 5: the right to liberty and security of person
- Article 6: the right to fair and independent hearings
- Article 8: the right to respect for private and family life, home and correspondence
- Article 9: the right of respect for religion, belief, etc.
- Article 10: the right of freedom of expression
- Article 14: the right not to be discriminated against in the recognition of the Articles.

The articles can be downloaded from the Internet from the Department of Health website (www.doh.gov.uk/humanrights).

NHS organisation

NHS trusts were established under the NHS and Community Care Act 1990 to provide secondary (hospital) care in the NHS. Under the National Health Service (Primary Care Act 1997), the Health Act 1999, Health and Social Care Act 2001, primary care groups, subsequently given trusts status, and care trusts have been established to organise community and primary care services and commission secondary services. (In Wales local health groups were replaced by Local Health Boards in 2003.) Funds are given to these primary care trusts to arrange for the provision of secondary services for patients in the catchment area. New strategic health authorities replaced the commissioning health authorities in England from April 2002.

GP contracts

General practitioners are mainly self-employed practitioners who have a contract for the provision of services, though increasingly salaried GP posts are being set up.

There is a significant difference between a person being an employee in contrast to a provider of services. An employee is covered by the vicarious liability of the employer (see below) and therefore would not have to pay personally compensation for harm arising from negligence committed in the course of employment. In contrast a self-employed person has to take out his or her own insurance cover. Where the self-employed person is also an employer then he or she will also be vicariously liable for any negligence of his or her employee. Thus a general practitioner who employs practice nurses and receptionists must ensure that they have employer's liability insurance cover as well as cover in respect of their own actions. The Medical Defence Union and the Medical Protection Society provide cover for their members.

The professional first aider

Accountability – criminal, civil, employer's and professional

When a patient dies or suffers harm as a result of failures by professional staff, then it is likely that various legal proceedings will be held to establish accountability and whether a criminal offence has occurred. Case study 1 illustrates a situation where there is an investigation following an incident where a patient died as a result of being given incorrect first aid. The situation will be explored to illustrate the criminal, civil, disciplinary and professional proceedings which could take place.

CASE STUDY 1
Accountability. First aid incorrectly administered

Primrose, a nurse, arrives at the scene, and notices that first aid is being incorrectly provided by Brian, a paramedic: he is performing inadequate chest compressions (far too slow). What action should Primrose take? Unfortunately Dennis, the patient, dies.

Coroner

In the case of an unexpected death, the death will have to be reported to the coroner. The statutory duty of the coroner is to establish the identity of the deceased and how, where and when the deceased came by his death; and the particulars, for the time being required by the Registration Acts, to be registered concerning the death. The coroner cannot make a finding that any person is criminally responsible for the death. However he/she can adjourn the inquest and ask the police and crown prosecution service to consider criminal proceedings.

Criminal proceedings

Health professionals can be found guilty of manslaughter if they have acted with such gross negligence in carrying out their professional work that their actions amount to a criminal act. This was the ruling by the House of Lords in the case of R. v Adomako (1994) where an anaesthetist was held guilty of manslaughter after a patient had died on the operating table. In the situation in Case study 1 it will be a question of fact as to whether Brian, the person administering the first aid treatment, acted with gross negligence and whether that incorrect treatment caused the death of the patient, Dennis. In a crown court jury trial, the jury would have to be satisfied beyond reasonable doubt both as to the gross negligence and the fact it caused the death. In addition, the nurse's failure to take appropriate action would be investigated, and if this amounted to gross negligence and a causative effect of Dennis's death, this too could be the subject of criminal proceedings.

Road traffic offences

Health professionals, as well as facing potential prosecution for gross negligence, are of course also subject to all the criminal laws of the country and could face prosecution for health and safety offences and road traffic offences. It has been of concern to ambulance drivers as to whether they were exempt from the road traffic offence of speeding when going to the scene of an accident or taking a patient to hospital. Many forces have been sent speeding notices when ambulances have been caught on camera. It was announced by the Department of Health in July 2004 that a new protocol for police forces had been agreed, which states that a fixed penalty notice can only be sent out to the ambulance trust if, on inspection of the photograph, blue lights cannot be seen flashing. It was thought that this would reduce the bureaucracy that ambulance staff have faced in the past when having to check whether the offending vehicle was on an emergency call. This checking was thought to cost the service £1 million a year.

Civil proceedings

All health professionals owe a duty of care to their patients. If a
patient has suffered harm as a result of negligence by a health
professional then the patient could bring an action for negligence
against that person or, more usually, the employer of that person.
The latter action is possible because of the doctrine of vicarious
liability which makes the employer liable for any harm caused by
the negligence of an employee who was acting in the course of his
employment. Any claimant would have to show that the employee
owed a duty of care which was broken when the employee failed to
follow a reasonable standard of care which caused the reasonably
foreseeable harm.

Duty of care

A duty of care exists between health professional and patient.
However, the law does not require any person to volunteer help, if
there is no preceding duty of care. This is discussed below.

Breach of the duty of care

To determine if there has been a breach of the duty of care, the
courts have used what has become known as the Bolam test. In the
case from which the test takes its name (Bolam v. Friern Barnet,
1957) Judge McNair said:

> *The standard of care expected is the standard of the ordinary skilled
> man exercising and professing to have that special skill.*

In Case study 1 it will be a question of fact determined as the result
of expert witnesses as to whether Brian, the paramedic, was in
breach of the duty of care he owed to the patient. Expert evidence
would also be required to establish whether any reasonable nurse,
following the approved standard of practice, would have acted in
the way that Primrose did.

Causation

To obtain compensation, the claimant must establish that the breach of duty caused the harm. In the scenario in Case study 1, it would have to be established that the breach of the duty of care by either Brian or Primrose (or both) caused the death of Dennis. This may be difficult since Dennis was clearly in a dangerous situation which could have caused death in itself.

CASE STUDY 2
Broken ribs

A nurse, Violet, is performing CPR in a first aid situation. Unfortunately she fractures the patient's ribs. Can the patient claim compensation?

In Case study 2, the crucial issues are: was Violet following the reasonable standard of care when she performed CPR and if not, did her failure cause the fractured ribs. Once again expert evidence would be required on both issues and if it were accepted by the court that CPR, no matter how carefully it was carried out, had an inevitable risk of fractured ribs, then it is unlikely that the patient would receive any compensation.

Harm

Harm is a vital element in obtaining compensation in an action for negligence. It may include loss or damage of property, pain suffering or death, and it may also include mental harm, such as post-traumatic stress disorder. It is important that those involved in a major accident take care to protect persons from the trauma which could cause serious mental illness.

CASE STUDY 3
Post-traumatic stress syndrome

There was a serious road accident involving several cars and a minibus carrying some young children. The police and ambulance crew who arrived on the scene failed to control the onlookers, one of whom, Mavis, had recognised a friend in the carnage and became hysterical. Subsequently, Mavis claimed that she had suffered from post-traumatic stress syndrome and her life was ruined. She is intending to sue the driver whose negligence caused the crash and if necessary the police and ambulance service.

In the case of Alcock v. Chief Constable South Yorkshire Police (1992), the House of Lords have ruled that, where a person is claiming for post-traumatic stress syndrome and has not been physically involved in the accident, the claimant must satisfy certain tests of proximity. In this case, people who were present at or watched the disaster at Hillsborough, where 95 people died (as a result of overcrowding in the stadium, allegedly due to negligence by the police), brought a claim in respect of post-traumatic stress syndrome. The House of Lords held that, in order to establish a claim in respect of psychiatric illness resulting from shock, it was necessary to show not only that such injury was reasonably foreseeable, but also that the relationship between the claimant and the defendant was sufficiently proximate. Proximity could include not only blood ties, but also ties of love and affection. The closeness would have to be proved in each individual case. The claimant would also have to show propinquity in time and space to the accident or its immediate aftermath. It was held that those claimants who viewed the disaster on television could not be said to be equivalent to being within sight and hearing of the event or its immediate aftermath.

In another case following the same incident, White and others v. Chief Constable of the South Yorkshire Police and others (1999), police officers sued for post-traumatic stress syndrome following the same disaster. The House of Lords decided that merely being an employee of the person/organisation responsible for the negligence did not automatically create sufficient proximity for the claimant to succeed in obtaining compensation for post-traumatic stress syndrome. The employee had to satisfy the usual rules of establishing proximity. To obtain compensation for psychiatric illness, a rescuer would have to show that he had objectively exposed himself to danger or reasonably believed that he was doing so. Rescuers were not entitled to claim compensation when they were not within the range of foreseeable physical injury and their psychiatric injury was caused by witnessing or participating in the aftermath of accidents which caused death or injury to others. The police therefore failed in their claim.

How do these cases apply to the scenario in Case study 3? In order to succeed in her claim against the negligent driver who caused the accident, Mavis would have to show that she was sufficiently proximate to the accident and to the injured person. If, for example, she had actually been in one of the cars which crashed, she would satisfy the proximity test. However, as an onlooker, it is unlikely that she would have a successful claim. Nor is her claim against the police or ambulance service likely to succeed. Mavis would have to prove that these organisations owed a duty of care to protect an onlooker from mental harm. The court would probably find that the primary duty of those organisations were to those involved in the crash.

If these elements of duty, breach, causation and harm can be established, then compensation is payable to the claimant. In the case of a death, there is a fixed statutory sum payable to the estate of the deceased (at present £10 000) but, in addition, those persons who were dependent upon the deceased, for example, wife and children, can claim in respect of their loss. Where the harm suffered by the patient is partly the result of their own failings, then if there are failures in the duty of care by a health professional, account would be taken of the patient's own responsibility in causing the harm which he/she has suffered. This is known as 'contributory negligence' and the judge would determine the extent to which any

Legal aspects of first aid
The professional first aider
317

compensation payable to the patient should be reduced to reflect the patient's fault.

In the scenario in Case study 1, there would appear to be a prima facie (at first sight) case of negligence by Brian, the paramedic, and possibly Primrose, the nurse. They owed Dennis a duty of care, they failed to follow a reasonable standard of care, if this failure caused the death of Dennis. However, compensation would probably be paid by their employer(s) on the basis of its vicarious liability for the negligence of an employee in the course of employment.

Negligence in communication

Failures in communicating are as much negligence as are failures in practice. It is imperative that every organisation providing health care has a regularly audited system to ensure good communications between staff and staff and between staff and patients, that records are properly kept and regularly referred to by staff. In a recent case, a mother notified a nursery that her five-month-old baby was allergic to cow's milk. An assistant gave the baby a cereal which contained milk protein and the baby died. An Inquest jury found that the baby died from neglect. The parents have declared their intention of suing the nursery (Fresco, 2003).

Future changes in compensation for clinical negligence

There are at the present time discussions taking place over whether a statutory scheme for compensation in clinical cases should be introduced which could include no-fault compensation (i.e. it would not have to be established that there was a breach of the duty of care), mediation, compensation calculated according to a tariff and the payment of structured settlements (Department of Health, 2001a). A further consultation paper was published in 2003 (Department of Health, 2003) and, at the time of writing, a white paper or draft legislation is awaited.

Disciplinary proceedings

The employer of the person whose actions have caused harm would be entitled to take disciplinary action against the employee. There is an implied term in a contract of employment that an employee will act with reasonable care and skill and obey reasonable instructions. In Case study 1, an investigation would have to take place and, if it was established that an NHS employee failed to ask the necessary questions or follow the correct procedure, then steps within the disciplinary procedure from an oral warning to dismissal on the ground of gross misconduct could take place.

Professional conduct proceedings

Any registered health professional would also face professional conduct proceedings which could lead to him or her being struck off the register. The actions of the nurse would be reported to the NMC which has the power to investigate the situation and, if considered appropriate, to hold a Conduct and Competence hearing. Similar professional conduct proceedings can be held by the Health Professions Council in respect of any practitioner registered with the HPC.

Expanded role

CASE STUDY 4
Emergency at an airport

Robert has a cardiac arrest at an airport. There is an automated external defibrillator on the wall. Rachel is the nurse on duty. She has not been trained to use the defibrillator but has watched colleagues use them. In this emergency can Rachel use the defibrillator?

Legal aspects of first aid
The professional first aider
319

In the scenario in Case study 4, Rachel is bound by her code of professional conduct and must work within her capacity. However, in an emergency situation where someone's life is at stake, it is a question of balancing the possibility of her saving Robert's life by using equipment she is not trained to use against the risk that he will die without that equipment. Clearly, if certain activities are reasonably foreseeable, it would be advisable to ensure that the health professional is trained in advance. Where health practitioners take on work as an expanded role they must ensure that the same standard of care is provided as would have been available if the person who had originally performed that activity had done it. It is no defence to say to a patient, 'I am sorry that you were harmed, but a staff nurse rather than a doctor undertook that activity and she did not have the training to take the appropriate action'.

Nurse prescribing

CASE STUDY 5
Expanded role

Rose, an emergency nurse, prescribes and administers aspirin. A patient suffers a severe anaphylactic reaction and dies.

In the situation in Case study 5, the prescribing and administering practice nurse has the responsibility of ensuring that the patient is safe. She should only give a medicine where she knows it is safe to do so. In addition, she should ensure that the patients have all the information necessary for them to be safe. Her training should ensure that she knows what medicines she is competent to prescribe and administer, that she knows the contraindications for each medicine and the appropriate dosages and she knows the limits of her competence and when she needs to seek further advice. The administration of aspirin without completing any checks about allergies would only be justified if the benefits of its administration outweighed the possibility of an anaphylactic reaction. This is unlikely to be so.

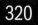
Initially community nurses and health visitors were given statutory powers to prescribe provided that they had had the necessary additional training. In February 2000 prescribing powers were given to nurses employed by a doctor on the medical list (i.e. GP) and also to nurses working in Walk-in Centres, defined in the regulations as: 'A Centre at which information and treatment for minor conditions is provided to the public under arrangements made by or on behalf of the Secretary of State'. As a result of the recommendations of the interim Crown Report (Department of Health, 1998) there are now statutory requirements (Amendment Order, 2000) for patient group directions under which nurses and other specified health professionals can prescribe. Further information can be obtained from Chapter 28 in the author's book (Dimond, 2004). The Final Crown Report (Department of Health, 1999) recommended that there should be statutory changes to enable health professions other than doctors to be identified and trained as independent or dependent prescribers. Legislation to progress these recommendations was contained in Section 63 of the Health and Social Care Act 2001 which amends the Medicines Act 1968.

Further developments in extending prescribing powers came into force on 1 April 2002. A statutory instrument (Amendment Order, 2002) laid down arrangements for a registered nurse and who is recorded in the register as qualified to order drugs, medicines and appliances from the Extended Formulary to prescribe products listed in the Extended Formulary. Schedule 3A of the statutory instrument sets out the substances which may be prescribed, administered or directed for administration by extended formulary nurse prescribers. The Schedule also sets out the conditions for such prescription or administration. The list includes antibiotics, analgesics and vaccines. Full details are published in the British National Formulary (BNF).

In November 2002 the NMC (Nursing and Midwifery Council, 2002) issued guidance on standards for the extension of independent prescribing by its registered practitioners. It sets out the standards and content of the programme for extended nurse prescribing and supplementary prescribing, and also the areas, knowledge and competencies required to underpin the practice of prescribing.

It could be argued that, since it is reasonably foreseeable that a patient might go into anaphylaxis following the administration of a drug by a nurse, then the nurse should be eligible and trained to prescribe and administer life-saving adrenaline (epinephrine).

Department of Health proposals

On 16 April 2002, the Department of Health published proposals to give nurses and pharmacists further prescribing powers to cover some chronic conditions. The proposals were implemented in 2003 and enable appropriately trained nurses and pharmacists to prescribe for such conditions as asthma, diabetes, high blood pressure and arthritis. Prescriptions for inhalers, hormone replacement therapy and anticoagulants are included.

In the situation in Case study 5, the nurse will have to show that she had the legal powers to prescribe and administer the drug that she gave to the patient, that she was following the reasonable standard of care in so doing, that she knew the necessary action to take following an allergic reaction and that she was not therefore acting illegally or negligently. When a nurse undertakes expanded role activities, she/he must follow the standard which could reasonably have been expected from the health professional who would usually have performed that role.

Multidisciplinary working

Unification of administration is not necessarily a guarantee of cooperation and coordination. Key working and team working depend upon each member of the team appreciating the role that others play in patient care. The law itself does not recognise any rule of team liability: each member of the team is personally and professionally accountable for his or her actions (Wilsher v. Essex Area Health Authority, 1986). Failures in communication can often lead to harm occurring to the patient and the Health Service Commissioners reports show that poor communications are often one of the main reasons why complaints arise.

The volunteer first aider

No legal duty to volunteer

Any claimant who is seeking compensation for alleged negligence
has to prove that a duty of care existed and that the defendant (or
employee of the defendant) was in breach of that duty of care (see
above). However, the law does not require people to volunteer help
and, unless there is a pre-existing duty, such as health
professional/patient, teacher/pupil, then there would be no legal
liability for failing to volunteer. That is the situation in law.
However, the Nursing and Midwifery Council expects its registered
practitioners to volunteer assistance as part of its code of
professional conduct. Paragraph 8.5 states:

*In an emergency, in or outside the work setting, you have a professional
duty to provide care. The care provided would be judged against what
could reasonably be expected from someone with your knowledge,
skills and abilities when placed in those particular circumstances.*

The nurse who failed to volunteer help could therefore not be held
legally liable in the civil courts for failing to act; she could, however,
face proceedings for fitness to practise. Where the nurse has
volunteered help in such a situation, it is unlikely that her employer
would accept any responsibility for her actions, i.e. would not be
vicariously liable (see above) and therefore the nurse would have to
rely on personal insurance cover in the event of any action being
brought against her. This cover, known as cover for Samaritan
actions, is provided by some professional associations. Professional
indemnity insurance cover is recommended by the NMC for its
registered practitioners (Nursing and Midwifery Council, 2002).

Standards of care in volunteering

While there is no legal duty to volunteer help, once that duty has
been assumed then there is a duty to take reasonable care of the

Legal aspects of first aid
The volunteer first aider
323

patient and failure to follow that standard if it led to additional harm suffered by the patient could lead to liability of the volunteer. In this situation it is unlikely that the employer would consider the volunteer's actions as being in the course of employment, and so the doctrine of vicarious liability would not apply and the volunteer would be reliant upon any Good Samaritan insurance cover that he or she had.

What standard of care should be followed by the volunteer?

The standard applied to the untrained volunteer is the standard of the ordinary person in the street: once known as 'the man on the Clapham omnibus'. In a case involving help at a race course by the St John Ambulance Brigade the judge applied the standard of the reasonable St John Ambulance officer (see Case study 6).

CASE STUDY 6

Case 1 Cattley v St John Ambulance Brigade QBD 25 November 1989 (Griffiths, 1990)

The St John Ambulance Brigade were sued by the person helped by two of their members on the grounds that they had caused the victim further harm. The person claiming compensation was 15 at the time of the accident. He had been competing in a motorcycle scramble for school boys. He came off his bike and was treated at the track by two brigade members. He suffered from cracked ribs and also compression fractures of the sixth and seventh dorsal vertebrae which had damaged the spinal cord and caused incomplete paraplegia. He claimed that the spinal injury was aggravated by the negligent examination and treatment offered him by the St John Ambulance personnel in the period immediately after the fall. It was alleged that he had been lifted to his feet, causing further damage to his already injured spinal cord.

The question arose: was there a duty of care owed and if so what was the standard? The Judge found no difficulty in holding that there was a duty of care and he held that the standard should be an adaptation of the Bolam test (Bolam v. Friern Barnet, 1957). Did the first aider act in accordance with the standards of the ordinary skilled first aider exercising and professing to have the special skills of a first aider?

In applying this test the judge rejected the evidence of the boy and his father and held that all the evidence pointed to the fact that at all times the first aiders had acted in accordance with the ordinary skill to be expected of a properly trained first aider. The claim was therefore rejected.

CASE STUDY 7
Volunteering help

Ada, a staff nurse in Out Patients, is walking to work when she hears a huge crash and realises that a car has driven into a motorbike. She is not trained in first aid but realises that the motorcyclist is in danger of dying unless an emergency tracheotomy was performed. The ambulance has been called but there is a likelihood that the casualty will die if the procedure is not undertaken promptly. She decides to try and help him but in so doing she causes his death. What is her legal liability?

In Case study 7, there was no legal duty placed upon Ada to assist the victim, but she had a professional duty under her code of professional conduct. The NMC suggests that in fulfilling her professional responsibilities:

The care provided would be judged against what could reasonably be expected from someone with your knowledge, skills and abilities when placed in those particular circumstances (Para. 8.5).

However, Ada has no first aid skills, she did her best, but was that sufficient in law? Expert evidence would be given about what could have been expected from a registered nurse who had no first aid skills in that set of circumstances. If she is found to have failed in providing a reasonable standard of care, then any claimant for compensation would still have to establish that it was what Ada did which caused the death and not the underlying condition of the patient. If Ada is sued successfully, her employer would not be vicariously liable for her actions as they were not carried out in the course of her employment. This means that she would have to rely upon insurance cover provided by a professional association or a private scheme.

Patients' rights

Right to services/drugs/operations

There is no absolute right to receive NHS services. The Secretary of State has a responsibility to provide reasonable services under the NHS Act 1977. There are certain services, however, which there is a statutory duty to provide: these include the provision of primary medical services, so that everyone is entitled to be placed upon a list of a general practitioner unless they have been violent.

The Secretary of State has a statutory duty under NHS legislation to provide a comprehensive National Health Service to meet all reasonable requirements, which covers both prevention and treatment and specifically requires a number of services to be provided. However, there have been a series of cases where the courts have held that provided the Secretary of State has fulfilled his/her statutory duty to provide a comprehensive National Health Service to meet all reasonable requirements and, provided there is no obvious evidence of irrational or unreasonable setting of priorities, then the courts will not be involved in the determination of the allocation of resources.

Thus, in the inevitable situation where resources are finite and demand outmatches supply, providers and commissioners of services have to weigh priorities. Examples of when individual patients have sought to enforce the statutory duty to provide services, and the courts have refused to intervene, include a case where patients sued the Secretary of State and other health organisations because they had waited too long for hip operations. They failed in their claim (R. v Secretary of State for Social Services, 1979). In another case, Mrs Walker failed to obtain a declaration that heart surgery should be carried out on her child (R. v Central Birmingham Health Authority, 1987). More recently, Jamie Bowen, a child suffering from leukaemia, was refused by the purchasers a course of chemotherapy and a second bone marrow transplant on the grounds that there was only a very small chance of the treatment succeeding and therefore it would not be in her best interests for the treatment to proceed. The Court of Appeal upheld the decision of the health authority (R. v. Cambridge HA, 1995).

Cases succeeding on grounds of failure to provide services

More recently, however, there have been several cases where the courts have upheld the right of an individual patient to access services. The first was in relation to the failure of a health authority to permit a drug for multiple sclerosis to be prescribed in its catchment area (R. v. North Derbyshire Health Authority, 1997). The health authority decided that it would not enable Beta Interferon to be prescribed for patients in its catchment area, since it was not yet proven to be clinically effective for the treatment of multiple sclerosis. A sufferer from multiple sclerosis challenged this refusal of the Health Authority and succeeded on the grounds that the health authority had failed to follow the guidance issued by the Department of Health (NHS Executive Letter EL (95)97). In the second case, a health authority refused to fund treatment for three transsexuals who wished to undergo gender reassignment (North West Lancashire Health Authority v. A, D, and G, 1999). The transsexuals sought judicial review of the health authority's refusal and the judge granted an order quashing the authority's decision and the policy on which it was based. The health authority then took the case to the Court of Appeal but lost its appeal. The Court of Appeal held that while the precise allocation and weighting of priorities is a matter for the judgment of the Authority and not for the court, it is vital for an Authority:

a. to assess accurately the nature and seriousness of each type of illness and

b. to determine the effectiveness of various forms of treatment for it and

c. to give proper effect to that assessment and that determination in the formulation and individual application of its policy.

The Authority failed to treat transsexualism as an illness, and its policy amounted to a 'blanket policy' against funding treatment for the condition because it did not believe in such treatment. There was no evidence that it genuinely considered individual exceptions. The court, however, held in respect of the human rights arguments that Article 3 and Article 8 of the European Convention on Human Rights (see above) did not give a right to free healthcare and did not apply to this situation, where the challenge is to a health authority's allocation of finite funds. Nor were the patients victims of discrimination on the grounds of sex.

Provision of ambulance services

In a recent case (Kent v. Griffiths and Others, 1998), the Court of Appeal held that, although the ambulance service owed no duty to the public at large to respond to a telephone call for help, once a 999 call had been accepted, it was arguable that the ambulance service did have an obligation to provide the service for a named individual at a specified address. Subsequently, the Court of Appeal dismissed an appeal by the London Ambulance Authority that it should pay the victim £362 377 (Kent v. Griffiths and Others, 2000). The facts of the case are shown below in Case study 8.

CASE STUDY 8

Case 2 Ambulance slow to arrive

A doctor called an ambulance for a woman who was asthmatic at 4.27 p.m. on 16 February 1991. The standards recommended were that the ambulance should come within 14 minutes. The husband phoned again at 4.39 p.m. and was told they would be there within 7 to 8 minutes. The doctor phoned at 4.55 p.m. and was told it would be a couple of minutes. The ambulance arrived at 5.05 p.m., 38 minutes after the first call. (A record prepared by a member of the crew indicated that it had arrived after 22 minutes.) During the journey, the claimant was given oxygen, but on the way suffered a respiratory arrest with tragic consequences, including serious memory impairment, change of personality and miscarriage. The judge found that the record of the ambulance's arrival had been falsified. The Court of Appeal refused to strike out the case as disclosing no reasonable cause of action for negligence, but held that the case should continue to trial.

Consent: living wills; autonomy; mentally incapacitated adult

It is a basic principle of the common law that a mentally competent adult has the right to give or refuse consent to treatment (Re MB (an adult: medical treatment), 1997). Even if the mentally competent adult requires life-saving treatment, that person has the right to refuse. The only requirement is that there should be clear evidence of the mental competence of the adult. Thus, where a tetraplegic patient was dependent upon a ventilator she was entitled to ask for it to be switched off (Re B, 2002). Two psychiatrists confirmed that she had the requisite mental capacity. The following tests of mental capacity were used by the Court of Appeal in a case where a pregnant woman refused to have a Caesarean section because she suffered a needle phobia (Re MB (an adult: medical treatment), 1997).

A person lacks the capacity if some impairment or disturbance of mental functioning renders the person unable to make a decision whether to consent to or to refuse treatment. That inability to make a decision will occur when:
- The patient is unable to comprehend and retain the information which is material to the decision, especially as to the likely consequences of having or not having the treatment in question
- The patient is unable to use the information and weigh it in the balance as part of the process of arriving at the decision.

Mental incapacity

Where a person lacks the mental capacity to make a decision, then action must be taken in his or her best interests (Re F (mental patient: sterilisation), 1990). There have been proposals for legislation to provide a statutory framework for decision making on behalf of mentally incapacitated adults (Lord Chancellor's Office, 1999). In Scotland, an Adults with Incapacity (Scotland) Act 2000 has come into force, but the rest of the UK still has to rely upon common law powers to act in the best interests of a mentally incapacitated adult. The Mental Capacity Act 2005 is due to come into force in April 2007.

Living will

CASE STUDY 9
An advanced refusal

Ambulance men were summoned to a house by a neighbour following a cardiac arrest. On arrival they were told by the wife that her husband had completed an advanced refusal and would not want any resuscitation. There was clearly a dispute between the wife and the neighbour. They were shown a piece of paper by the wife, which appeared to be an advanced refusal by the husband to have resuscitation in the event of a cardiac arrest. It was signed and witnessed and dated 9 months before. What action should they take?

In the situation in Case study 9, the ambulance men would have to form a view over the validity of the advanced refusal signed by the man. If there were any doubt over its validity it would be preferable for them to save the man's life. Advanced refusals are being placed on a statutory basis by the Mental Capacity Act 2007.

Children

Young persons of 16 and 17 have a statutory right under the Family Law Reform Act 1969 to give consent to treatment. Treatment is widely defined and covers surgical, medical and dental treatment, anaesthesia and diagnostic procedures. Where a young person gives consent, then there is no requirement for the parents also to consent. Where the young person is unable to give consent, then parents can consent on the child's behalf until the child is an adult at 18 years.

Although young persons and children below 16 do not have a statutory right to give consent, they do have a right recognised at common law by the House of Lords in the Gillick case (Gillick v. W. Norfolk and Wisbech Area Health Authority, 1986), provided that they have the mental capacity to understand the information and the risks involved, i.e. that they are 'Gillick competent'. For the 16 and 17 year old there is a presumption of capacity which can be rebutted, for the child under 16 the requisite mental capacity must be established.

Child refusing treatment

While a young person of 16 and 17 has a statutory right to give consent, and a child of any age has a right recognised at common law to give consent if Gillick competent, the principle has been set by the Court of Appeal that, if life-saving treatment is necessary and in the best interests of the child, then a person under 18 years cannot give a valid refusal. Thus an anorexic girl of 16 years was compelled to receive treatment. In case 3 shown in Case study 10, a young girl of 15 years was compelled to have a heart transplant against her will.

CASE STUDY 10
Case 3 Refusing a transplant (Re M, 1999)

A girl of 15 years refused to consent to a transplant which was needed to save her life. She stated that she did not wish to have anyone else's heart and she did not wish to take medication for the rest of her life. The hospital, which had obtained her mother's consent to the transplant, sought leave from the court to carry out the transplant.

The court held that the hospital could give treatment according to the doctor's clinical judgement, including a heart transplant. The girl was an intelligent person whose wishes carried considerable weight, but she had been overwhelmed by her circumstances and the decision she was being asked to make. Her severe condition had developed only recently and she had had only a few days to consider her situation. While recognising the risk that for the rest of her life she would carry resentment about what had been done to her, the court weighed that risk against the certainty of death if the order were not made.

Confidentiality

CASE STUDY 11
Confidentiality

Mohammed was involved in a road traffic accident and is being treated in hospital. While still not fully recovered he wishes to take his own discharge from hospital because he wishes to return to his job as a taxi driver. He has been advised by his doctor that he should not be driving a car. However, the doctor knows that he is likely to ignore this advice.

All health professionals are bound by a duty of confidentiality in relation to information learnt about the patient and given to them in confidence. This duty derives from many sources:

- trust relationship between patient and professional
- implied term in the contract of employment
- statutory provisions, such as the Data Protection Act 1998
- professional codes of conduct
- duty of care to the patient may include a recognition that the duty of care includes the safekeeping of confidential information.

The law recognises many exceptions to this duty which are:
- the consent of the patient
- disclosure in the interests of the patient, e.g. to the multidisciplinary team
- the requirement of the court for information to be given
- several Acts of Parliament recognise a situation where confidential information can be passed on, e.g. informing the police about a road accident in which there has been personal injury; information passed under the Prevention of Terrorism legislation; notification of infectious diseases under public health legislation
- disclosure in the public interest, e.g. reporting concerns about child protection; where serious harm to the physical or mental health of the patient or another person is feared.

In the situation in Case study 11, there is a clear danger to public safety in Mohammed continuing to drive and the doctor should be protected under the need to act in the interests of the safety of the public if he were to report Mohammed to the Driving Licence Authority. The doctor should, of course, first attempt to persuade Mohammed to stay in hospital and not to drive, warning him that he commits a criminal offence if he drives when advised that he is medically unfit to do so, and alerting him to the fact that the doctor himself could report it, if Mohammed himself failed to stop driving until he was medically fit.

Complaints

A new complaints scheme for the NHS came into force in July 2004 (Department of Health, 2001b). It follows research over several years on the scheme established in 1996 following the Wilson Report into complaints (Department of Health, 1994). It places statutory duties upon NHS trusts and primary care trusts to investigate complaints according to a strict time limit and places upon the Healthcare Commission (CHAI) responsibility for setting up panels for the second stage of the complaints procedure. The jurisdiction of the Health Service Commissioner (Ombudsman) is retained to investigate further if the complainant is still dissatisfied.

Legal aspects of first aid
Health and safety laws
333

Health and safety laws

First aid regulations

The Health and Safety (First-Aid) Regulations were passed in 1981 and have been published by the Health and Safety Commission with an Approved Code of Practice and Guidance (The Health and Safety (First-Aid) Regulations, 1981). They replace earlier regulations, enacted in 1960, which required the provision of first aid boxes. The replacement regulations were far more extensive in their definition of the duties of employers in relation to first aid at work and cover the following topics:

definition of first aid

duty of employer to make provision for first aid

duty of employer to inform employees of the arrangements made in connection with first aid

duty of self-employed person to provide first aid equipment

power to grant exemptions

cases where regulations do not apply but other regulations do.

In the Guidance, Appendix 1 provides an assessment of first aid needs checklist and Appendix 2 the definition of competencies following first aid training which successful candidates should have obtained following training.

First aid is defined as:

a. in cases where a person will need help from a medical practitioner or nurse, treatment for the purpose of preserving life and minimising the consequences of injury and illness until such help is obtained, and

b. treatment of minor injuries which would otherwise receive no treatment or which do not need treatment by a medical practitioner or nurse.

The employer has a duty to provide, or ensure that there are provided, such equipment and facilities as are adequate and appropriate in the circumstances for enabling first aid to be rendered to employees if they are injured or become ill at work. In addition, the employer must provide or ensure that there is provided such number of suitable persons as is adequate and appropriate in the circumstances for rendering first aid to employees if they are injured or become ill at work. A person is not suitable unless he had undergone such training and has such qualifications as the Health and Safety Executive may approve for the time being in respect of that case of class of case and such additional training, if any, as may be appropriate in the circumstance of that case.

Where a qualified first aider is absent in temporary and exceptional circumstances it is sufficient if the employer appoints, throughout the period of any such absence, a person or ensures that a person is appointed, to take charge of the situation relating to an injured or an ill employee who will need help from a medical practitioner or nurse and the equipment and facilities required above. If the appointment of a person in charge is the preferred option having regard to the nature of the undertaking, the number of employees at work and the location of the establishment, then this could take the place of the appointment of first aiders. Guidance on the employer's duty covers the assessment of first aid need and the relevant factors which should be taken into account in making that assessment. The guidance also covers the first aid materials, equipment and facilities which may be appropriate, including the provision of first aid containers, additional first aid materials, including travelling first aid kits, and first aid rooms. Guidance on first aid personnel includes a table setting out the suggested numbers of first aid personnel to be available at all times.

The duty of the employers to provide information for employees states:

An employer shall inform his employees of the arrangements that have been made in connection with the provision of first aid, including the location of the equipment, facilities and personnel.

Legal aspects of first aid
Health and safety laws
335

Manual handling

. . . .

> CASE STUDY 12
> A lifting nightmare
>
> Mary cares for her elderly father who is severely disabled with
> multiple sclerosis. She has support from social services three
> times a day. She has been informed that they wish a hoist to
> be installed and will not allow their care staff to handle her
> father manually. Both she and her father object to the use of
> the hoist and Mary says that she has never had difficulties in
> raising and lifting him on her own. Her father says that it is
> contrary to his human rights to be forced to be hoisted.

All health professionals in primary care are subject to health and
safety legislation. The main duties placed on both employer and
employee are set out in the Health and Safety at Work Act 1974.
These statutory duties are supplemented by regulations. These
include the Manual Handling regulations on which guidance is
provided by the Health and Safety Executive (Health and Safety
Executive, 1992). In addition to the statutory duties there are
implied terms in the contract of employment that an employee will
take reasonable care of the health and safety of employees. In the
situation in Case study 12, clearly social services or the agency
providing the care assistants have a statutory duty and also a
contractual duty to ensure that reasonable care is taken of the
health and safety of employees and therefore that where manual
handling can be reasonably avoided, then that is done and that
other steps are taken to reduce the risk of harm from any remaining
manual handling. It would appear a reasonable request to use a
hoist. It is unlikely that Mary and her father would succeed in
arguing that they had a right under the European Convention of
Human Rights for a hoist not to be used, since with skilful use
hoisting should not be seen as degrading or inhuman treatment
under Article 3. In a case in East Sussex where relatives and clients
objected to the use of hoists, claiming that it was a breach of their

human rights, the judge held that there was not a human right not to be hoisted, but nor was there a human right for the carers to insist upon a hoist being used: it all depended upon the risk assessments of the individual circumstances (A and B v. East Sussex County Council, 2003).

Case 4 shown in Case study 13 indicates the problems for ambulance officers in moving patients from their homes.

CASE STUDY 13

Case 4 Ambulance men and manual handling (King v. Sussex Ambulance NHS Trust, 2002)

King, an ambulance technician, suffered serious injuries carrying an elderly patient down the stairway of his home. He and his colleague had taken the patient down the stairway, which was narrow and steep, in a carry chair. He had been injured when forced for a brief moment to bear the full weight of the chair.

The judge found in favour of the ambulance technician, holding that the employers were in breach of Council Directive (90/269; Article 3(2)) and the Manual Handling Regulations, and that the employers had acted negligently by discouraging employees in circumstances such as those in this particular case from calling the fire brigade to take patients from their homes.

Sussex Ambulance NHS Trust appealed against the finding. The Court of Appeal held that the NHS trust was not liable either under the Directive or under the Manual Handling Regulations. There was nothing to suggest that calling the fire brigade would have been appropriate in the case. The evidence showed that such an option was rarely used because it had to be carefully planned, took a long time and caused distress to the patient. There might be cases where calling the fire brigade would be appropriate, but that would depend on the seriousness of the problem, the urgency of the case and the

Legal aspects of first aid
Health and safety laws
337

actual or likely response of the patient or his/her carers and the fire brigade.

King had failed to show that giving that possibility more emphasis in training would have avoided his injuries. The ambulance service owed the same duty of care to its employees as did any other employer. However, the question of what was reasonable for it to do might have to be judged in the light of its duties to the public and the resources available to it when performing those duties. While the risks to King had not been negligible, the task that he had been carrying out was of considerable social utility.

Furthermore, Sussex Ambulance NHS Trust had limited resources so far as equipment was concerned. There was no evidence of any steps that the trust could have taken to prevent the risk and the only suggestion made was that it should have called on a third party to perform the task for it. Since calling the fire brigade was not appropriate or reasonably practicable for the purpose of the directive and the regulations, the Sussex Ambulance NHS Trust had not shown a lack of reasonable care. Accordingly, it had not acted negligently.

Manual handling is only one of many areas of health and safety laws relevant to health care and each trust and PCT should ensure that there is an identified officer who ensures compliance with risk assessment and management principles, the medical devices regulations, the reporting of incidents, injuries and diseases and other legislation. The National Patient Safety Agency will require reports of incidents and hazards to be notified so that they can ensure that these incidents do not occur elsewhere (Dimond, 2005).

Record keeping

It goes without saying that record keeping of the professional activities that have taken place is essential. Where the first aider is an employee, this should be part of the treatment and care provided, to indicate to others the action that has been taken, so that if the patient is moved elsewhere there is documentary evidence over what has been done. However, there would be advantages in the volunteer who helps out in an emergency situation keeping a record of what action he or she has taken in case at some future stage there were to be an investigation into the incident.

Conclusion

Unfortunately this chapter is but a superficial description of some of the laws that are relevant to those involved in first aid, but it is hoped that it will provide a path through the legal maze to more detailed knowledge.

References

A and B v. East Sussex County Council (The Disability Rights Commission an interested party) [2003] EWHC 167 (Admin)

Alcock v. Chief Constable S. Yorks. Police 1992 2 AC 310 HL

Bolam v. Friern Barnet HMC [1957] 1 WLR 582; [1957] 2 All ER 118

Department of Health (1994) Being Heard. The report of a review committee on NHS Complaints Procedures May 1994. Department of Health, London

Department of Health (1998) Review of Prescribing, Supply and Administration of Medicines: a report on the supply and administration of medicines under Group Protocols. April

Department of Health (1999) Review of Prescribing, Supply and Administration of Medicines Final Report (Crown Report) March 1999. Department of Health, London

Department of Health (2001a) Press release 2001/0313. New Clinical Compensation Scheme for the NHS. 20 July

Department of Health (2001b) Reforming the NHS Complaints Procedure: a listening document DoH September 2001; The National Health Service (Complaints) Regulations 2004 SI 2004 No 1768

Department of Health (2003) Making Amends. A consultation paper setting out proposals for reforming the approach to clinical negligence in the NHS CMO. June

Department of Health (2004) Green light for ambulances on speeding fine problem. 2 July

Dimond B (2004) Legal Aspects of Nursing, 4th edn. Pearson Education, London

Dimond B (2005) Legal Aspects of Health and Safety. Quay Publications, Dinton, Wiltshire

Fresco A (2003) Milk baby died after nursery's neglect. The Times, 29 January

Gillick v. W. Norfolk and Wisbech Area Health Authority [1986] 1 AC 112

Griffiths G (1990) Cattley v. St John's Ambulance Brigade QBD 25 November 1989 unreported. Discussed in article in Modern Law Review, 53: 255

Health and Safety Executive (1992) Manual Handling Guidance on Regulations. HMSO, London

Kent v. Griffiths and Others, The Times Law Report 23 December 1998

Kent v. Griffiths and Others (no 2), The Times Law Report 10 February 2000; [2000] 2 All ER 474

King v. Sussex Ambulance NHS Trust [2002] EWCA 953; Current law August 2002 408

Lord Chancellor's Office (1999) Making Decisions: The Government's Proposals for Decision Making on Behalf of the Mentally Incapacitated Adult. October. Stationery Office, London

NHS Executive Letter: EL (95)97

North West Lancashire Health Authority v. A, D, and G [1999] Lloyds Law Reports Medical page 399

Nursing and Midwifery Council (2002) Extended independent nurse prescribing and supplementary prescribing NMC 25/2002 12 November

Nursing and Midwifery Council (2004) New clause added to the NMC code of professional conduct: standards for conduct, performance and ethics

R. v. Adomako [1994] 2 All ER 79

R. v. Cambridge HA ex parte B [1995] 2 All ER 129

R. v. Central Birmingham Health Authority ex parte Walker (1987) 3 BMLR 32; The Times 26 November 1987

R. v. North Derbyshire Health Authority [1997] 8 Med L R 327

R. v. Secretary of State for Social Services ex parte Hincks and others. 29 June 1979 (1979) 123 Solicitors Journal 436

The Health and Safety (First-Aid) Regulations (1981) Health and Safety Commission with an Approved Code of Practice and Guidance

White and others v. Chief Constable of the South Yorkshire Police and others [1999] 1 All ER 1

Wilsher v. Essex Area Health Authority [1986] 3 All ER 801 CA

Further reading

Dimond B (2002) *Legal Aspects of Patient Confidentiality*. Quay Publications, Dinton, Wiltshire

Dimond B (2002) *Legal Aspects of Pain Management*. Quay Publications, Dinton, Wiltshire

Dimond B (2003) *Legal Aspects of Consent*. Quay Publications, Dinton, Wiltshire

Dimond B (2004) *Legal Aspects of Nursing*, 4th edn. Pearson Education, London

Dimond B (2005) *Legal Aspects of Medicine*. Quary Publications, Dinton, Wiltshire

Health and Safety Commission (1992) *Manual Handling Regulations and Approved Code of Practice*. HMSO, London

Hurwitz B (1998) *Clinical Guidelines and the Law*. Radcliffe Medical Press, Oxford

Kennedy I, Grubb A (2000) *Medical Law and Ethics*, 3rd edn. Butterworth, London

McHale J, Gallagher A (2004) *Nursing and Human Rights*. Butterworth-Heinemann, London

McHale J, Tingle J (2001) *Law and Nursing*. Butterworth-Heinemann, London

Pitt G (2000) *Employment Law*, 4th edn. Sweet and Maxwell, London

Selwyn N (2000) *Selwyn's Law of Employment*, 11th edn. Butterworth, London

Wilkinson R, Caulfield H (2000) *The Human Rights Act: a Practical Guide for Nurses*. Whurr Publishers, London

Alk Abello (2005) **Intructions for the administration of adrenaline via the EpiPen auto-injector**. Hungerford: Alk Abello Ltd

Allison K, Porter K (2004) Consensus on the pre-hospital approach to burns patient management. **Emerg Med J**, 21: 112–114

American Academy of Pediatrics (2000) **Pediatric Education for prehospital professionals**. USA: American Academy of Pediatrics

American College of Surgeons (1997) **Advanced Trauma Life Support for Doctors Instructor Course Manual**. American College of Surgeons, Chicago

American College of Surgeons (2004) **Advanced Trauma Life Support for Doctors**, 7th edn. American College of Surgeons, Chicago

American Heart Association (AHA) in Collaboration with ILCOR (2000) Guidelines 2000 for Cardiopulmonary Resuscitation and Emergency Cardiovascular Care – An International Consensus on Science. **Resuscitation**, 46: 1–448

Ashworth H, Cubison T, Gilbert P et al (2001) Treatment before transfer: the patient with burns. **Emerg Med J**, 18: 349–351

B (Consent to treatment: Capacity) The Times Law Report 26 March 2002

Bahr J, Klingler H, Panzer W et al (1997) Skills of lay people in checking the carotid pulse. **Resuscitation**, 35: 23–26

Baskett P, Nolan J, Parr M (1996) Tidal volumes that are perceived to be adequate for resuscitation. **Resuscitation**, 31: 231–234

Benditt D, Goldstein M (2002) Fainting. **Circulation**, 106: 1048–1050

Berg M, Idris A, Berg R (1998) Severe ventilatory compromise due to gastric distension during cardiopulmonary resuscitation. **Resuscitation**, 36: 71–73

Bissing J, Kerber R (2000) Effect of shaving the chest of hirsute subjects on transthoracic impedance to self-adhesive defibrillation electrode pads. **Am J Cardiol**, 86(5): 587–589, A10

Bjork R, Snyder B, Campion B, Loewenson R (1982) Medical complications of cardiopulmonary arrest. **Arch Intern Med**, 142: 500–503

Bosworth C (1997) **Burns Trauma**: Management and Nursing Care. Baillière Tindall, London

Bowman F, Menegazzi J, Check B, Ducket T (1995) Lower esophageal sphincter pressure during prolonged cardiac arrest and resuscitation. **Ann Emerg Med**, 26: 216–219

Brenner B, Chavda K, Karakurum M et al (1999) Circadian differences among 4096 patients presenting to the emergency department with acute asthma. **Acad Emerg Med**, 6: 523

Brignole M, Alboni P, Benditt D et al (1999) Guidelines on management (diagnosis and treatment) of syncope. **Eur Heart J**, 22: 1256–1306

British Heart Foundation (2005) Factfile 05/2000 **Chest pain – is it angina?** Accessed from www.bhf.org April 2005

British Red Cross (2003) **Practical First Aid**. Dorling Kindersley, Middlesex

British Thoracic Society & Scottish Intercollegiate Guidelines Network (BTS & SIGN) (2004) **Update to the British Guideline on the Management of Asthma**. www.sign.ac.uk

British Thoracic Society & Scottish Intercollegiate Guidelines Network (BTS & SIGN) (2005) **The BTS/SIGN British Guideline on the Management of Asthma**. www.brit-thoracic.org.uk

Butcher M (2001) Burns trauma assessment. **Nurse 2 Nurse**, 12(1): 9–10

Centers for Disease Control (1988) Update: universal precautions for prevention of transmission of human immunodeficiency virus, hepatitis B virus and other blood-borne pathogens in healthcare settings. **MMWR**, 37: 377–388

Chameides L, Berlin P, Cummins R et al (2000) New guidelines for first aid in American Heart Association (2000) Guidelines 2000 for Cardiopulmonary Resuscitation and Emergency Cardiovascular Care: International Consensus on Science. **Circulation**, 102(8): I-77–85

Chan E et al (1998) **Bedside Critical Care Manual**. Philadelphia: Hanley and Belfus

Chestnutt M, Prendergast T (2004) **Current medical diagnosis and treatment**. Columbus OH: McGraw-Hill Companies

Cilcot J, Howell S, Kemeney A et al (1999) **The Effectiveness of Surgery in the Management of Epilepsy**. Guidance Note for Purchasers InterDec Report 15/1999. Trent Institute for Health Services Research

Coats T, Davies G (2002) Pre-hospital care for road traffic casualties. **BMJ**, 324: 1135–1138

Cockerell OC, Hart YM, Sander JWAS et al (1994) The cost of epilepsy in the United Kingdom: an estimation based on the results of two population based studies. **Epilepsy Research**, 18: 249–260

Committee on Trauma of the American College of Surgeons (1997) **Advanced Life Support Instructor Manual**. Chicago: American College of Surgeons

Cummins R, Hazinski M, Kerber R et al (1998) Low-energy biphasic waveform defibrillation: evidence-based review applied to emergency cardiovascular care guidelines: a statement for healthcare professionals from the American Heart Association Committee on Emergency Cardiovascular Care and the Subcommittees on Basic Life Support, Advanced Life Support and Paediatric Life Support. **Circulation**, 97: 1654–1667

Department of Health (2005a) Heatwave: **Plan for England**. Department of Health, London

Department of Health (2005b) Tetanus www.dh.gov.uk accessed 14/06/05

Department of Trade & Industry (1999) **Home and Leisure Accident Report: Summary of 1998 Data**. HMSO, London

Department of Trade & Industry (1999) **Home and Leisure Accident Surveillance System, 1978-1997**. Department of Trade & Industry, London

Diabetes UK (2002) **Hypoglycaemia**. Diabetes UK, London

Eberle B, Dick WF, Schneider T et al (1996) Checking the carotid pulse check: diagnostic accuracy of first responders in patients with and without a pulse. **Resuscitation**, 33: 107–116

Electricity Association (2004) **Watch it! Guidance for Emergency Services Carrying Out a Rescue in the Vicinity of Overhead Lines, Substations and Other Electrical Equipment**. Electrical Association, London

Epilepsy Action (2004) Epilepsy Information: **First Aid For Seizures** www.epilespy.org.uk

European Resuscitation Council (ERC) (1998) **Periarrest arrhythmias: management of arrhythmias associated with cardiac arrest**. European Resuscitation Council Guidelines for Resuscitation. Oxford: Elsevier

European Resuscitation Council (ERC) (1998) **European Resuscitation Guidelines for Resuscitation**. Brussels: European Resuscitation Council

Evans R, Burke D (1995) **Key topics in accident and emergency medicine**. BIOS, Oxford

Evans R, Burke D (2001) **Key topics in accident and emergency medicine**, 2nd edn. BIOS, Oxford

F (mental patient: sterilisation) [1990] 2 AC 1

Flesche CW, Brewer S, Mandel LP et al (1994) The ability of health professionals to check the carotid pulse. **Circulation**, 90: 1–288

Fowler A (2003) The assessment and classification of non-complex burns injuries. **Nursing Times**, 99(25): 46–47

GISSI (1998) Ten year follow-up of the first megatrial testing thrombolytic therapy in patients with acute myocardial infarction: results of the GISSI study. **Circulation**, 98: 2659–2665

Graveling A, Warren R (2004) Hypoglycaemia and driving in people with insulin-treated diabetes: adherence to recommendations for avoidance. **Diabetic Medicine**, 21(9): 1014–1019

Guildner CW (1976) Resuscitation – opening the airway: a comparative study of techniques for opening an airway obstructed by the tongue. **J Am Coll Emerg Phys**, 5: 588–590

Haley C, McDonald R, Rossi L et al (1989) Tuberculosis epidemic among hospital personnel. **Infect Control Hosp Epidermiol**, 10: 204–210

Handley A, Handley J (1995) The relationship between the rate of chest compression and compression:relaxation ratio. **Resuscitation**, 30: 237–241

Henderson J (2005) Respiratory support of infants with bronchiolitis related apnoea: is there a role for negative pressure? **Archives of Disease in Childhood**, 90(3): 224–225

Hettiaratchy S, Dziewulski P (2004a) ABC of burns: Introduction. **BMJ**, 328: 1366–1368

Hettiaratchy S, Dziewulski P (2004b) ABC of burns: pathophysiology and types of burns. **BMJ**, 328: 1427–1429

Hettiaratchy S, Papini R (2004) ABC of burns: initial management of a major burn: 2 – assessment and resuscitation. **BMJ**, 329: 101–103

Hinds CJ, Watson D (1999) ABC of intensive care: circulatory support. **BMJ**, 318: 1749–1752

Hudspith J, Rayatt S (2004) ABC of burns: First aid and treatment of minor burns. **BMJ**, 328: 1487–1489

Hugdel DW, Hendricks C (1988) Palate and hypopharynx: sites of inspiratory narrowing of the upper airway during sleep. **Am Rev Respir Dis**, 138: 1542–1547

Idris A, Wenzel V, Banner M, Melker R (1995) Smaller tidal volumes minimise gastric inflation during CPR with an unprotected airway. **Circulation**, 92(suppl 1): 1759 Abstract

Idris AH, Florete OG Jr, Melker RJ et al (1996) Physiology of ventilation, oxygenation and carbon dioxide elimination during cardiac arrest.

Jevon P (2002) **Advanced cardiac life support**. Oxford: Butterworth-Heinemann

Jones G, Endacott R, Crouch R (2003) **Emergency Nursing Care**. Greenwich Medical Media Ltd, London

Keech P (2004) **Practical Guide to First Aid**. Lorenz Books, London

Kuckelkorn R, Schrage N, Keller G, Redbrake C (2002) Emergency treatment of chemical and thermal eye burns. **Acta Ophthalmologica Scandinavica**, 80(1): 4–10

Kyle M, Wallace A (1951) Fluid replacement in burnt children. **Br J Plastic Surg**, 3: 194

Lawes E, Baskett P (1987) Pulmonary aspiration during unsuccessful cardiopulmonary resuscitation. **Intens Care Med**, 13: 379–382

London Energy (2004) **Safety in your home and garden**. London Energy, London

Lund C, Bowder N (1944) Estimation of area of burns. **Surgery, Gynaecology & Obstetrics**, 79: 352–358

M (Medical Treatment: Consent) [1999] 2 FLR 1097

MB (an adult: medical treatment) (1997) 38 BMLR 175 CA; 2 FLR 426

Maier G, Tyson G Jr, Olsen C et al (1984) the physiology of external cardiac massage: high impulse cardiopulmonary resuscitation. **Circulation**, 70: 86–101

Marcus R (1988) Surveillance of health care workers exposed to blood from patients infected with the human immunodeficiency virus. **N Engl J Med**, 319: 1118–1123

Mejicano G, Maki D (1998) Infections acquired during cardiopulmonary resuscitation: estimating the risk and defining strategies for prevention. **Ann Intern Med**, 129: 813–828

Melker RJ (1985) Recommendations for ventilation during cardiopulmonary resuscitation: a time for change? **Crit Care Med**, 13(pt 2): 882–883

Melker RJ, Banner MJ (1985) Ventilation during CPR: two rescuer standards re-appraised. **Ann Emerg Med**, 14: 197

Mellesmo S, Pillgram-Larsen J (1995) Primary care of amputation injuries. **JEUR**, 8: 131–135

Meningitis Research Foundation (2005) www.meningitis.org

National Institute for Clinical Excellence (2002) **Press Release: 2002/026 NICE launches National Clinical audit of epilepsy-related death**. www.nice.org.uk

National Safety Council (1999) Injury Facts, 1999 Edition. Itasca, 111: National Safety Council: 1999: 9–15. National Safety Council, USA

National Society for Epilepsy (2004) **Epilepsy: what to do when someone has a seizure**. National Society for Epilepsy, Bucks

NMC (2002) **The NMC code of professional conduct: standards for conduct, performance and ethics**. NMC, London

NMC (2005) www.nmc-uk.org accessed 14 March 2005

Nunez A, Mora J (2004) Organisation of Medical Care in Acute Stroke: Importance of a Good Network. **Cerebrovascular Diseases Ischaemic Stroke**, 17(suppl 1): 113–123

Nurhantari Y, Asano M, Nushida H et al (2002) Accidental hanging by a sweater: an unusual case. **American Journal of Forensic Medicine & Pathology**, 23(2): 199–201

Nursing Times (2005) **Facts – Croup**. 101(3): 30

Office for National Statistics (1998) **Mortality statistics**

Paradis N, Martin G, Goetting M et al (1989) Simultaneous aortic, jugular bulb, and right atrial pressures during cardiopulmonary resuscitation in humans: insights into mechanisms. **Circulation**, 80(suppl 2): 11496 Abstract

Piazza M, Chirianni A, Picciotto L et al (1989) Passionate kissing and microlesions of the oral mucosa: possible role in AIDS transmission. **JAMA**, 261: 244–245 letter

Prescription Only Medicines (Human Use) Amendment Order (2000) SI 2000 No 1917

The Prescription Only Medicines (Human Use) Amendment Order (2002) Statutory Instrument 2002 No 549

Pumphrey R (2004) **Novartis Foundation Symposium**, 275: 116–132

Ramrakha P, Moore K (2004) **Oxford Handbook of Acute Medicine**, 2nd edn. Oxford University Press, Oxford

Rees J, Kanabar D (2000) **ABC of Asthma**, 4th edn. BMJ Books, London

Resuscitation Council (UK) (2000) **Advanced Life Support Provider Manual**, 4th edn. London: Resuscitation Council (UK)

Resuscitation Council (UK) (2000a) **Resuscitation Guidelines 2000**. London: Resuscitation Council (UK)

Resuscitation Council (UK) (2000b) **Cardiopulmonary Resuscitation: Guidance for Clinical Practice and Training in Hospitals**. London: Resuscitation Council (UK)

Resuscitation Council (UK) (2001) **Guidance for Safer Handling during Resuscitation in Hospitals**. Resuscitation Council (UK), London

Resuscitation Council UK (2003) **European Paediatric Life Support Course Provider Manual**. Resuscitation Council UK, London

Resuscitation Council (UK) & British Heart Foundation (2003) **Resuscitation for the citizen**. London: Resuscitation Council

Robertson C, Fenton O (2000) **Management of severe burns**. In Driscoll P, Skinner D, Earlam R (eds) ABC of Major Trauma, 3rd edn. BMJ Books, London

Rodrigo G, Rodrigo C, Hall J (2004) Acute asthma in adults: a review. **Chest**, 125(3): 1081–1102

Royal Life Saving Society (RLSS) and the Royal Society for the Prevention of Accidents (ROSPA) (2005) **Water safety factsheet**. RLSS, Broom

Royal Society for the Prevention of Accidents (2001) **First Aid Hints for Burns and Scalds**. www.rospa.co.uk

Ruben HM, Elam JO, Ruben AM (1961) Investigation of upper airway problems in resuscitation. Studies of pharyngeal X-rays and performance by lay men. **Anesthesiology**, 22: 271–279

Safar P (1958) Ventilatory efficiency of mouth to mouth respiration: airway obstruction during manual and mouth to mouth artificial ventilation. **JAMA**, 167: 335

Safar P (1974) Pocket mask for emergency artificial ventilation and oxygen inhalation. **Crit Care Med**, 2: 273–276

Scarfone R (2005) Controversies in the treatment of bronchiolitis. **Current Opinion in Pediatrics**, 17(1): 62–66

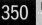

Scottish & Southern Energy (2001) **Treatment for electric shock. In Safety and Environmental Manual**. Scottish & Southern Energy, Scotland

Sharvon S (2000) **Handbook of epilepsy treatment**. Blackwell, Oxford

Sheridan R (2003) Burn care: results of technical and organisational progress. **JAMA**, 290(6): 719

SIGN (2003) **Diagnosis and management of epilepsy in adults**. Scottish Intercollegiate Guidelines Network, Edinburgh

Smith G (2003) **ALERT: Acute Life Threatening Events Recognition and Treatment**. University of Portsmouth, UK

St John Ambulance, St Andrew's Ambulance, British Red Cross (2002) **First Aid Manual**, 8th edn. Dorling Kindersley, London

Stone B, Chantler P, Baskett P (1998) The incidence of regurgitation during cardiopulmonary resuscitation: a comparison between the bag-valve-mask and laryngeal mask airway. **Resuscitation**, 38: 3–6

Stroke Association (2005) www.stroke.org.uk

Taylor K (2001) The management of minor burns and scalds in children. **Nursing Standard**, 16(11): 45–52

Trim J (2005) Performing a comprehensive physiological assessment. **Nursing Times**, 100(50): 38–42

Watkins P (2003) **ABC of Diabetes**, 5th edn. BMJ Books, London

Wenzel V, Idris A, Banner M et al (1994) The composition of gas given by mouth-to-mouth ventilation during CPR. **Chest**, 106: 1806–1810

World Health Organization (2002) Department of Injuries and Violence Prevention. www.who.int

www.eguidelines.co.uk (February 2005) Guidelines – summarising clinical guidelines for primary care

Wyatt J, Illingworth R, Clancy M et al (2005) **Oxford Handbook of Accident & Emergency Medicine**. Oxford University Press, Oxford

Further reading

Al-balkhi A, Klonin H, Marinaki K et al (2005) Review of treatment of bronchiolitis related apnoea in two centers. **Archives of Disease in Childhood**, 90(3): 288–291

Ambrose J, Fuster V (1997) Can we predict future acute coronary events in patients with stable coronary artery disease? (editorial; comment). **JAMA**, 277: 343–344

Angeras M, Brandberg A, Falk A, Seeman T (1992) Comparison between sterile saline and tap water for the cleaning of acute traumatic soft tissue injuries. **Europ J Surgery**, 158: 6–7, 347–350

Appleton M, Jerreat L (1995) **Hypoglycaemia. Nursing Standard**, 10(5): 36–42

Belvis R, Cocho D, Marti-Fabregas J (2005) Benefits of a prehospital stroke code system: feasibility and efficacy in the first year of clinical practice in Barcelona, Spain. **Cerebrovascular Diseases**,19(2): 96–101

Bennett G, Moody M (1995) **Wound Care for Health Professionals**. Chapman & Hall, London

Bolli G et al (1983) Abnormal glucose counter-regulation in insulin-dependent diabetes mellitus. Interaction of anti-insulin antibodies and impaired glucagon and epinephrine secretion. **Diabetes**, 32: 134–141

Boyne L (2001) Meningococcal infection. **Nursing Standard**, 16(7): 47–55

Brown S, Betts T, Crawford P et al (1998) Epilepsy needs revisited: a revised epilepsy needs document for the UK. **Seizure**, 7: 435–446

Buck D, Baker G, Jacoby A et al (1997) Patients' experiences of injury as a result of epilepsy. **Epilepsia**, 38: 439–444

Budnick L (1984) Bathtub related electrocutions in the United States, 1979–1982. **JAMA**, 252: 918–920

Bui T, Delgado C, Simon H (2002) Infant seizures not so infantile: first-time seizures in children under six months of age presenting to the ED. **American Journal of Emergency Medicine**, 20(6): 518–520

Cahill C, Lloyd-Davies V, Hartington K (2000) **Trauma in hostile environments**. In Driscoll et al (eds) ABC of Major Trauma. BMJ Books, London

Chang K, Tseng M, Tan T (2004) Pre-hospital delay after acute stroke in Kaohsiung, Taiwan. **Stroke**, 35(3): 700–704

Chelliah A, Mark R (2004) Hypoglycaemia in elderly patients with diabetes mellitus: causes and strategies for prevention. **Drugs & Aging**, 21(8): 511–530

Chesebro J, Rauch U, Fuster V, Badimon J (1997) Pathogenesis of thrombosis in coronary artery disease. **Haemostasis**, 27(suppl 1): 12–18

Collier M (1996) Trauma injury nursing in A & E. Wound Care Supplement. **Nursing Times**, 92(20)

Department of Health (2005) **Tetanus**. www.dh.gov.uk accessed 14/06/05

Department of Trade & Industry (1999) **Home and Leisure Accident Report: Summary of 1998 Data**. HMSO, London

Department of Trade & Industry (1999) **Home and Leisure Accident Surveillance System, 1978–1997**. Department of Trade & Industry, London

Docherty B (2002) Cardiorespiratory physical assessment for the acutely ill. **Brit J Nursing**, 11(11): 750–758

Driscoll T, Harrison J, Steenkamp, M (2004) Review of the role of alcohol in drowning associated with recreational aquatic activity. **Injury Prevention**, 10(2): 107–113

Evans R, Burke D (2001) **Key topics in accident and emergency medicine**, 2nd edn. BIOS, Oxford

Fasol R, Sheena I, Zilla A (1989) Vascular injuries caused by anti-personnel mines. **J Cardiovasc Surg**, 30: 467–472

Fisher J (2004) Out-of-hospital cardiopulmonary arrest in children with croup. **Pediatric Emergency Care**; 20(1): 35–36

Forbes T, Carson M, Harris K et al (1995) Skeletal muscle injury induced by ischaemia-reperfusion. **Can J Surg**, 38: 56–63

Gallagher G, Rae C, Kinsella J (2000) Treatment of pain in severe burns. **American J Clin Dermatology**, 1(6): 329–335

Garcia-Sanchez V, Gomez M (1999) Electric burns: high and low tension injuries. **Burns**, 25: 357–360

Goodacre S, Kelly A-M, Kerr D (2004) Potential impact of interventions to reduce times to thrombolysis. **Emerg Med J**, 21: 625–629

Gowens P, Davenport R, Kerr J et al (2003) Survival from accidental strangulation from a scarf resulting in laryngeal rupture and carotid artery stenosis: the 'Isadora Duncan syndrome'. A case report and review of literature. **Emergency Medicine Journal**, 20: 391–393

Gray K, Cheng E, Pegg S (2004) Hot cooking oil burns: a 20 year experience. **J Burn Care & Rehabilitation**, 25(2): 205–210

Greaves I, Porter K (eds) (1999) **The Principles and Practice of Immediate Care**. Arnold, London

Greaves I, Dyer P, Porter K (1995) **Handbook of Immediate Care**. WB Saunders, London

Greaves I et al (2001) **Trauma Care Manual**. Arnold, London

Harulow S (1995) Assessment of burn injuries. **Emergency Nurse**, 2(4): 19–22

Hasibeder W (2003) Drowning. **Current Opinion in Anaesthesiology**, 16(2): 139–145

Hayes C (2004) Clinical skills: practical guide for managing adults with epilepsy. **Br J Nursing**, 13(7): 380–386

Hubbuck K (2003) Treatment of children with severe burns. **Lancet**, 362: S44

Husum H (1999) Effects of early prehospital life support to war injured: the battle of Jalalabad, Afghanistan. **Prehospital Disaster Medicine**, 14: 75–80

Iung O, Wade F (1963) The treatment of burns with ice water, Phisohex, and partial hypothermia. **Industrial Med Surg**, 32: 365–370

Johnson R, Richard R (2003) Partial-thickness burns: identification and management. **Advances in Wound Care**, 16(4): 178

Khaw P, Shah P, Elkington A (2004) **ABC of Eyes**. BMJ Books, London

Kubiak T, Hermanns N, Schreckling H et al (2004a) Assessment of hypoglycaemia awareness using continuous glucose monitoring. **Diabetic Medicine**, 21(5): 487–490

Kubiak T, Kuhr B, Inselmann D et al (2004) Reversible cognitive deterioration after a single episode of severe hypoglycaemia: a case report. **Diabetic Medicine**, 21(12): 1366–1367

Lavy J, Koay C (1996) First aid treatment of epistaxis: are the patients well informed? **J Accid Emerg Med**, 13: 193–195

Lawrence E (2004) Diagnosis and Management of Migraine Headaches. **South Med J**, 97(11): 1069–1077

Lip G, Brodie M (1992) Sudden death in epilepsy: an avoidable outcome? **J R Soc Med**, 85: 609–11

Lipton R, Bigal M, Steiner T et al (2004) Classification of primary headaches. **Neurology**, 63: 427–435

Ludman H (2002) **ABC of Otolaryngology**, 4th edn. BMJ Publishing, London

Lunetta P, Smith G, Penttila A, Sajantila A (2004) Unintentional drowning in Finland 1970-2000: a population-based study. **International Journal of Epidemiology**, 33(5): 1053–1063

Lyden P, Rapp K, Babcock T, Rothcock J (1994) Ultra-rapid identification, triage, and enrolment of stroke patients into clinical trials. **J Stroke Cerebrovasc Dis**, 4: 106–107

Mason A (1994) **First Aid**. Ward Lock, London

Masoorli S (1997) Consult Stat: These bandages can impair an IV infusion. **RN** 60(5): 69

Matsuyama T, Okuchi K, Seki T, Murao Y (2004) Prognostic factors in hanging injuries. **American Journal of Emergency Medicine**, 22(3): 207–210

McGarry G, Moulton C (1993) The first aid management of epistaxis by accident and emergency department staff. **Arch Emerg Med**, 10: 298–300

McLaren E, Somerville J (1988) Early warning signs of hypoglycaemia in ambulant diabetics. **Practical Diabetes**, 5(5): 207–208

Midwinter I, Hodgson D, Yardley M (1999) Paediatric epiglottitis: the influence of the Haemophilus influenzae b vaccine, a ten-year review in the Sheffield region. **Clinical Otolaryngology & Allied Sciences**, 24(5): 447–448

Moon R, Long R (2002) Drowning and near-drowning. **Emergency Medicine**, 14(4): 377–386

Morse S, Hardwick W, King W (1997) Fatal iron intoxication in an infant. **South Med J**, 90: 1043–1047

Moserova J, Behounkova E (1975) Subcutaneous temperature measurements in thermal injury. **Burns**, 1: 267–268

Moulton C, Yates D (1999) **Lecture notes on emergency medicine**. Blackwell Science, Oxford

Murray V (2000) **Chemical incidents**. In Driscoll P, Skinner D, Earlam R (eds) ABC of Major Trauma, 3rd edn. BMJ Books, London

National Institute for Clinical Excellence (2003) **Epilepsy: diagnosis and management of epilepsy in children and adults**. www.nice.org.uk

Neufeld M, Vishne T, Chistik V et al (1999) Life-long history of injuries related to seizures. **Epilepsy Res**, 34: 123–127

Nikolic S, Micic J, Atanasijevic T et al (2003) Analysis of neck injuries in hanging. **American Journal of Forensic Medicine & Pathology**, 24(2): 179–182

Odeh M (1991) The role of reperfusion-induced injury in the pathogenesis of the crush syndrome. **N Engl J Med**, 324: 1417–1422

Ofeigsson J, Mitchell R, Patrick R (1972) Observations on the cold water treatment of cutaneous burns. **J Pathology**, 108: 145–150

O'Neill D, LeGrove A (2003) Monitoring critically ill patients in accident and emergency. **Nursing Times**, 99(45): 32–35

Passaretti D, Billmire D (2003) Management of paediatric burns. **J Craniofacial Surgery**, 14(5): 713–718

Petrasek P, Shervanti H, Walker P (1994) Determinants of ischaemic injury to skeletal muscle. **J Vasc Surg**, 19: 623–630

Purdue G, Layton T, Copeland C (1985) Cold injury complicating burn therapy. **J Trauma**, 25: 167–168

Quan L, Cummings P (2003) Characteristics of drowning by different age groups. **Injury Prevention**, 9(2): 163–168

Resuscitation Council (UK) (2001) **Guidance for Safer Handling during Resuscitation in Hospitals**. Resuscitation Council (UK), London

Resuscitation Council (UK) (2005) **Resuscitation Guidelines 2005** Resuscitation Council (UK), London

Resuscitation Council (UK) (2006) **Statement on the use of Automated External Defibrillators (AEDs) until re-programming to be compliant with Guidelines 2005; Updated April 2006.** Resuscitation Council (UK), London

Resuscitation Council (UK) (2006a) **Statement on teaching paediatric life support to laypeople.** Resuscitation Council (UK), London

Ricketts S, Kimble F (2003) Chemical injuries: the Tasmanian burns unit experience. **ANZ J Surgery**, 73(1–2): 45–48

Riordan M, Rylance G, Berry K (2002) Poisoning in children: general management. **Arch Dis Child**, 87: 392–396

Riordan M, Rylance G, Berry K (2002a) Poisoning in children 4: household products, plants and mushrooms. **Arch Dis Child**, 87: 403–406

Riyat M, Quinton D (1997) Tap water as a wound cleansing agent in accident and emergency. **J Accident & Emergency Medicine**, 14(3): 165–166

Robertson C, Fenton O (2000) **Management of severe burns**. In Driscoll P, Skinner D, Earlam R (eds) ABC of Major Trauma, 3rd edn. BMJ Books, London

Rooney S, Hyde J, Graham T (2003) **Chest injuries**. In Driscoll P, Skinner D, Earlam R (eds) ABC of Major Trauma, 3rd edn. BMJ Books, London

Royal Society for the Prevention of Accidents (2001) **First Aid Hints for Burns and Scalds**. www.rospa.co.uk

Shirayama H, Ohshiro Y, Kinjo Y et al (2004) Acute brain injury in hypoglycaemia-induced hemiplegia. **Diabetic Medicine**, 21(6): 623–624

Sharvon S (2000) **Handbook of epilepsy treatment**. Blackwell, Oxford

Shulman A (1960) Ice water as primary treatment of burns: simple method of emergency treatment of burns to alleviate pain, reduce sequelae, and hasten healing. **JAMA**, 173: 1916–1919

Singer A, Mohammed M, Tortora G et al (2000a) Octylcyanoacrylate for the treatment of contaminated partial-thickness burns in swine: a randomised controlled experiment. **Acad Emerg Med**, 7: 222–227

Singer A, Thode J, McCain S (2000) The effects of epidermal debridement of partial-thickness burns on infection and reepithelialisation in swine. **Acad Emerg Med**, 7: 114–119

Strachan D, England J (1998) First aid treatment of epistaxis: confirmation of widespread ignorance. **Postgrad Med J**, 863: 113–114

Sunderland R, Fleming D (2004) Continuing decline in acute asthma episodes in the community. **Archives of Disease in Childhood**, 89(3): 282–285

Swain A, Dove J, Baker H (2003) **The spine and spinal cord**. In Driscoll P, Skinner D, Earlam R (eds) ABC of Major Trauma, 3rd edn. BMJ Books, London

Tan L, Calhoun K (1999) Epistaxis. **Otolaryngol Internist**, 83: 43–57

Tatum W, Liporace J, Benbadis S, Kaplan P (2004) Updates on the treatment of epilepsy in women. **Arch Internal Medicine**, 164(2): 137–145

Thorvaldsen P, Davidsen M, Bronnum-Hansen H, Schroll M (1999) Stable stroke occurrence despite incidence reduction in an aging population: stroke trends in the Danish monitoring trends and determinants in cardiovascular disease (MONICA) population. **Stroke**, 30: 2529–2534

Thorvaldsen P, Kuulasmaa K, Rajakangas A et al (1997) Stroke trends in the WHO MONICA project. **Stroke**, 28: 500–506

Turner J (2004) Prevention of drowning in infants and children. **Dimensions of Critical Care Nursing**, 23(5): 191–193

Wahlen M, Thierbach A (2002) Near-hanging. **European Journal of Emergency Medicine**, 9(4): 348–350

Westaby S (1985) **Wound care**. William Heinemann, London

Williams B (2004) In intensive care because he couldn't find an NHS dentist. Daily Mirror, Wednesday November 17

Williams G, Jiang J, Matchar D, Samsa G (1999) Incidence and occurrence of total (first-ever and recurrent) stroke. **Stroke**, 30: 2523–2528

Wilson S, Cook M (1998) Double bandaging of sprained ankles. **BMJ**, 317: 1722–1723

Wood B, Haque S, Weinstock A et al (2004) Pediatric stress-related seizures: conceptualization, evaluation, and treatment of nonepileptic seizures in children and adolescents. **Current Opinion in Pediatrics**, 6(5): 523–531

Yano K, Hosokawa K, Kakibuchi M et al (1995) Effects of washing acid injuries to the skin with water: an experimental study using rats. **Burns**, 21: 500–502

Young K, Okada P, Sokolove P et al (2004) A randomized, double-blinded, placebo-controlled trial of phenytoin for the prevention of early posttraumatic seizures in children with moderate to severe blunt head injury. **Annals of Emergency Medicine**, 43(4): 435–446

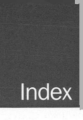

Index

Page numbers in *italics* refer to figures, tables or boxes.

R

S